300 MCQs
for the Duke Elder
Ophthalmology Exam

300 MCQs
for the Duke Elder Ophthalmology Exam

Anmol Patel
South Thames Deanery, UK

Dalia Abdulhussein
Northwest Thames Deanery, UK

Harkaran Kalkat
West Midlands Central Deanery, UK

Peng Yong Sim
Moorfields Eye Hospital, UK

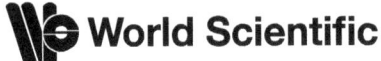

EW JERSEY • LONDON • SINGAPORE • BEIJING • SHANGHAI • HONG KONG • TAIPEI • CHENNAI • TOKYO

Published by

World Scientific Publishing Co. Pte. Ltd.
5 Toh Tuck Link, Singapore 596224
USA office: 27 Warren Street, Suite 401-402, Hackensack, NJ 07601
UK office: 57 Shelton Street, Covent Garden, London WC2H 9HE

British Library Cataloguing-in-Publication Data
A catalogue record for this book is available from the British Library.

300 MCQs FOR THE DUKE ELDER OPHTHALMOLOGY EXAM

Copyright © 2021 by World Scientific Publishing Co. Pte. Ltd.

All rights reserved. This book, or parts thereof, may not be reproduced in any form or by any means, electronic or mechanical, including photocopying, recording or any information storage and retrieval system now known or to be invented, without written permission from the publisher.

For photocopying of material in this volume, please pay a copying fee through the Copyright Clearance Center, Inc., 222 Rosewood Drive, Danvers, MA 01923, USA. In this case permission to photocopy is not required from the publisher.

ISBN 978-981-123-177-3 (hardcover)
ISBN 978-981-123-305-0 (paperback)
ISBN 978-981-123-178-0 (ebook for institutions)
ISBN 978-981-123-179-7 (ebook for individuals)

For any available supplementary material, please visit
https://www.worldscientific.com/worldscibooks/10.1142/12148#t=suppl

300 SBAs for the Duke Elder Prize Examination

Anmol Patel MBBS BSc (Hons) AICSM
Foundation Year 2 Doctor at Dartford and Gravesham NHS Trust

Dalia Abdulhussein MBBS BSc (Hons) AICSM
Academic Foundation Year 2 Doctor in Surgery at Imperial College London

Harkaran Kalkat MBBS BSc (Hons) AICSM
Foundation Year 2 Doctor at Sandwell and West Birmingham Hospitals NHS Trust

Peng Yong Sim BMedSci (Hons) MBChB (Hons) PGDip Clin Ed FHEA
ST3 Ophthalmology at Moorfields Eye Hospital

Senior Reviewers

Timothy Yap BMedSci (Hons) MA MBChB MRCP
Clinical Research Fellow (Ophthalmology)
Ophthalmology Specialist Trainee
Imperial College London, UK

Eduardo M. Normando MD PhD FEBO
Glaucoma Specialist
Clinical Senior Lecturer, Imperial College London
Honorary Consultant Ophthalmologist, Western Eye & Charing Cross Hospital
OPD Lead for CXH Ophthalmology
NWL Regional Undergraduate Education Lead
Honorary Senior Research Associate, UCL Institute of Ophthalmology, London, UK

Karl Mercieca MD PGCert FRCOphth FEBOS-GL
Consultant Ophthalmologist and Glaucoma Surgeon
Manchester Royal Eye Hospital, Manchester, UK
Honorary Senior Lecturer & Glaucoma Co-Lead, IOVS MSc Course, Manchester University, UK

Contents

300 SBAs for the Duke Elder Prize Examination		v
Senior Reviewers		vii
Introduction		xi
Chapter 1	Cornea and External Eye Disease Questions	1
Chapter 1	Cornea and External Eye Disease Answers	7
Chapter 2	Cataract Questions	15
Chapter 2	Cataract Answers	21
Chapter 3	Glaucoma Questions	29
Chapter 3	Glaucoma Answers	36
Chapter 4	Medical Retina and Vitreoretinal Surgery Questions	41
Chapter 4	Medical Retina and Vitreoretinal Surgery Answers	47
Chapter 5	Strabismus and Paediatric Ophthalmology Questions	53
Chapter 5	Strabismus and Paediatric Ophthalmology Answers	58
Chapter 6	Neuro-ophthalmology Questions	67
Chapter 6	Neuro-ophthalmology Answers	74
Chapter 7	Ocular Adnexal and Orbital Disease Questions	85
Chapter 7	Ocular Adnexal and Orbital Disease Answers	91
Chapter 8	Refractive Errors and Optics Questions	101
Chapter 8	Refractive Errors and Optics Answers	106
	Mock Exam Paper Questions	115
	Mock Exam Paper Answers	135

Introduction

What is the Duke Elder exam?

The Duke Elder prize exam is run by the Royal College of Ophthalmologists (RCOphth) annually. It is open to all UK medical undergraduates provided they have not graduated at the time of the examination. At the time of this publication, the 2-hour exam consists of 90 multiple choice questions (MCQs) in the single best answer (SBA) format where there are 4 options per question. Candidates are encouraged to attempt all questions, as there is no negative marking.

What is in the exam?

The exam tests knowledge in ophthalmology beyond that of the undergraduate curriculum. Consequently, candidates should expect a higher standard than that of their own university's undergraduate ophthalmology examination. There is currently limited specification of the exam syllabus by the RCOphth. The main emphasis is on clinical ophthalmology but other areas such as ocular physiology, anatomy, pathology, as well as genetics and socio-economic (e.g., epidemiology, world blindness, blind registration and driving legislation) relevant to ophthalmology may also be examined. The main 8 sections are outlined:

Topic	Brief Description Of Contents
Cornea and External Eye Disease	— Anatomy and refractive properties of cornea — Anatomy of conjunctiva, episcleral and sclera — Conditions related to these areas
Cataract	— Anatomy of the lens — Types of cataract — Management of cataract

(Continued)

(Continued)

Glaucoma	— Aqueous formation and drainage — Subtypes of glaucoma and their underlying pathology — Management of glaucoma
Medical Retina and Vitreoretinal Surgery	— Pathologies of the retina — Management of retinal conditions
Strabismus and Paediatric Ophthalmology	— Strabismus — Congenital ocular and orbital abnormalities
Neuro-ophthalmology	— Cranial nerve defects: CN III, IV and VI — Visual pathway and defects — Systemic conditions relevant to this
Ocular Adnexal and Orbital Disease	— Anatomy of the lid margin and orbit — Pathologies relating to these systems
Refractive Errors and Optics	— Basic concepts of optics — Refractive abnormalities

How should I prepare for the exam?

Ophthalmology in the undergraduate curriculum is often neglected and candidates should therefore expect more extensive preparation for the Duke Elder prize exam. For core reading material, it is important to consult the latest recommended reading list by the RCOphth and we recommend focusing more on practice questions, which will be of higher yield nearer to the exam.

In this book, we provide 200 practice questions in the SBA format (25 for each of the corresponding topics outlined above), followed by a 100-question mock test at the end. We suggest completing this mock test in 2 hours and 15 minutes to simulate exam conditions. Some topics are more exhaustive than others and where they are not covered in the practice questions, we have included these in the mock exam. We hope this book will serve as a valuable aid in your revision and we wish you every success for the exam.

Chapter 1 Cornea and External Eye Disease Questions

1) Which of the following statements regarding conjunctival anatomy is **FALSE**?
   A. The bulbar conjunctiva is continuous with corneal epithelium
   B. Blood supply is from the anterior ciliary artery
   C. Goblet cells are found in the conjunctival epithelium
   D. Accessory lacrimal glands are found in the conjunctival epithelium

2) Which of the following type of discharge is most commonly seen in chronic allergic conjunctivitis?
   A. Watery
   B. Mucoid
   C. Mucopurulent
   D. Moderately purulent

3) Which of the following statements regarding follicles in conjunctivitis is **TRUE**?
   A. They are seen in bacterial conjunctivitis
   B. They are subepithelial lymphoid germinal centres
   C. Histologically there are mature cells centrally and immature cells peripherally
   D. They are almost always abnormal in adults

4) A 20-year-old female presents with an acute unilateral red eye with watery discharge. On a systems review he has some dysuria and urinary frequency. On examination you note conjunctival follicles. Which of the following investigations would **NOT** be helpful in determining the cause of this?
   A. McCoy cell culture
   B. Direct immunofluorescence
   C. Polymerase chain reaction (PCR)
   D. Sabouraud agar

5) A mother has brought in her 6-day-old son, who is complaining of a red right eye with yellow discharge. On inspection, there is hyperpurulent discharge and severe eyelid oedema on the right eye. An ENT examination was normal. Which of the following organisms is most likely responsible for this clinical picture?
   A. Chlamydia trachomatis
   B. Herpes simplex virus (HSV)
   C. Staphylococcus aureus
   D. Neisseria gonorrhoea

6) A 32-year-old presents with redness and grittiness in her left eye. She is also complaining of a sore throat and a runny nose. On inspection, there is watery discharge and conjunctival hyperaemia. Which of the following is the most likely causative organism?
   A. HSV
   B. Adenovirus serovars 3, 4 and 7
   C. Coxsackie virus
   D. Molluscum contagiosum

7) A 54-year-old man presents with grittiness and a painless growth on his left eye. He normally resides in the Middle East. On inspection, there is a triangular ingrowth of conjunctival tissue over the limbus onto the cornea. Which of the following statements regarding this diagnosis is **TRUE**?
   A. It typically invades the Bowman layer of the cornea
   B. It tends to be temporal more often than nasal
   C. The most common cause is chemical damage to the eye
   D. Surgery is curative and associated with a low rate of recurrence

8) What is the average central corneal thickness?
   A. 510 μm
   B. 530 μm
   C. 550 μm
   D. 570 μm

9) Which of the following statements regarding the structure of the cornea is **FALSE**?
   A. The epithelium is stratified squamous non-keratinised
   B. The majority of corneal thickness is comprised of stroma
   C. The Descemet membrane is secreted by the endothelium
   D. The Bowman layer contains goblet cells

10) Which of the following organisms is **NOT** able to penetrate a healthy corneal epithelium?
    A. *Neisseria gonorrhoea*
    B. *Neisseria meningitidis*
    C. *Corynebacterium diphtheriae*
    D. *Staphylococcous aureus*

11) Which of the following infections is most likely to cause reduced corneal sensation?
    A. Herpes keratitis
    B. Bacterial keratitis
    C. Fungal keratitis
    D. Microsporidial keratitis

12) Which of the following statements regarding disciform keratitis is **FALSE**?
    A. It may be a hypersensitivity reaction to HSV antigen in the cornea
    B. Discomfort is milder than with epithelial keratitis
    C. It typically causes anterior uveitis
    D. Granulomatous precipitates underlie the oedema

13) A 43-year-old gentleman presents to his GP with an erythematous rash on his face that is causing pain around his eyes. On inspection, he has a well-demarcated vesicular rash on an erythematous base on the right side of his forehead, which does not cross the midline. His right eyelid is oedematous. There are also some lesions involving the side of the nose. Which of the signs in his presentation would confer a high risk of ocular involvement?
    A. Age
    B. Eyelid oedema
    C. Lesion on the side of nose
    D. Periocular pain

14) A 12-year-old boy is brought into the clinic with recent severe blurring of his vision. He has hearing aids but is otherwise well. On inspection, you note that he has a saddle-nose deformity and small, widely spaced teeth. Which ocular structure abnormality is likely to explain his visual symptoms?
    A. Retina
    B. Conjunctiva
    C. Corneal stroma
    D. Lens

15) Which of the following systemic conditions is the most common cause of peripheral ulcerative keratitis?
    A. Granulomatosis with polyangiitis
    B. Polyarteritis nodosa
    C. Systemic lupus erythematosus
    D. Rheumatoid arthritis

16) Which of the following may **NOT** cause neurotrophic keratopathy?
    A. Bell palsy
    B. HSV keratitis
    C. Diabetes mellitus
    D. Stroke

17) Bitot spots, keratomalacia, keratinisation and lustreless cornea are all signs of which disease?
    A. Sjögren syndrome
    B. Xerophthalmia
    C. Filamentary keratopathy
    D. Keratoconus

18) A 27-year-old presents with a continuous feeling of "something" in his eyes. Occasionally this is accompanied with discomfort to bright lights and redness. On examination there are well-demarcated filament-like lesions stained with rose Bengal seen on the corneal surface. Which of the following is important to enquire about in his history?
    A. Diet
    B. Contact lens wear
    C. Occupation
    D. Sun exposure

19) Which of the following statements regarding keratoconus is **TRUE**?
    A. Eye rubbing has no effect
    B. LASIK surgery may help
    C. Most patients often have a family history
    D. Presentation tends to be with unilateral progressive myopia and astigmatism

20) A 46-year-old female presents with gradual blurring of vision in both eyes, which is noted to be worse in the morning. An examination reveals the appearance of cornea guttata on Descemet membrane. Which of the following is the most likely diagnosis?
    A. François central cloudy dystrophy
    B. Fuchs endothelial corneal dystrophy
    C. Posterior polymorphous corneal dystrophy
    D. Congenital hereditary endothelial dystrophy

21) A 54-year-old woman presents with worsening vision in both eyes. She mentions that for the past month she has been feeling progressively worse and complains of abdominal pain, constipation, low mood and generalised aches. Which of the following may explain her reduced visual acuity?
    A. Lipid keratopathy
    B. Band keratopathy
    C. Spheroidal degeneration
    D. Salzmann nodular degeneration

22) A 19-year-old male is seen in an eye clinic. His background includes depression with psychosis, rigidity and tremor, which is under investigation. On a slit lamp examination, you note a brown-yellow zone of dusting in the cornea as well as scleral icterus. Which layer of the cornea are you likely to identify this in?
    A. Epithelium
    B. Bowman layer
    C. Stroma
    D. Descemet membrane

23) Which of the following is **NOT** a contraindication to ocular tissue donation?
   A. Death from an unknown cause
   B. Prior high-risk behaviour for HIV and hepatitis
   C. Corneal refractive surgery
   D. Prior treated brain cancer

24) Which of the following is a late complication of penetrating keratoplasty?
   A. Cystoid macular oedema
   B. Endophthalmitis
   C. Astigmatism
   D. Raised intraocular pressure (IOP)

25) A 60-year-old has attended eye casualty complaining of a gradually worsening persistent pain in his right eye, which radiates up to his brows and temple. Analgesia has not helped and the pain has been interfering with his sleep. He has no past medical history of note but has had right trabeculectomy surgery 4 weeks ago. Which of the following are you most likely to find on examination?
   A. Isolated patches of scleral oedema
   B. Oedema of the sclera, episclera, conjunctiva and adjacent cornea
   C. Localised area of necrosis extending outwards
   D. Diffuse scleral necrosis

Chapter 1

Cornea and External Eye Disease Answers

1) D

Conjunctiva is the transparent mucous membrane lining the anterior surface of the eye and the inner surface of the eyelids. It is divided into palpebral, forniceal and bulbar conjunctiva. Blood supply is from the anterior ciliary and palpebral arteries, both originating from the ophthalmic artery. The bulbar conjunctiva covers the anterior sclera and is continuous with corneal epithelium. Histologically it is divided into the following:

Histology	Contents
Epithelium	Goblet cells
Stroma	Accessory lacrimal glands of Krause and Wolfring
Conjunctiva-associated Lymphoid Tissue (CALT)	Lymphocytes and lymphatics

2) B

Conjunctival inflammation commonly results in discharge. The character of discharge often indicates the aetiology:

Discharge	Aetiology
Watery	Acute viral or acute allergic conjunctivitis
Mucoid	Chronic allergic conjunctivitis
Mucopurulent	Chlamydial or acute bacterial conjunctivitis
Moderately Purulent	Acute bacterial conjunctivitis
Severe Purulent	Gonococcal conjunctivitis

3) B

Follicles are subepithelial lymphoid germinal centres (central immature lymphocytes and peripheral mature cells), which are seen as slightly elevated lesions on the fornices. The most common causes are viral and chlamydial conjunctivitis. Other causes include hypersensitivity to topical medications. Small follicles are normal in adults when in fornices and at margins of the upper tarsal plate.

4) D

This describes a case of acute chlamydial conjunctivitis, which tends to occur in young sexually active patients. In female patients this would present with typical conjunctivitis symptoms and symptoms of chlamydial urethritis (e.g., dysuria, discharge). Investigations include PCR, Giemsa staining, direct immunofluorescence (to detect free elementary bodies), McCoy cell culture and enzyme immunoassay. Sabouraud agar is used to culture fungal organisms.

5) D

Neonatal conjunctivitis typically develops within the first month of life. The following organisms are most commonly implicated:

Organism	Features
Staphylococci	• Onset: end of first week • Mildly sticky eye
Herpes simplex virus	• Onset: 1–2 weeks • May have vesicles and features of encephalitis • Watery discharge
Chlamydia	• Onset: 1–3 weeks • Disseminated infection is more common than with others (rhinitis, pneumonitis, otitis) • Mucopurulent discharge
Neisseria	• Onset: first week • Hyperpurulent discharge

In this case Neisseria is likely to be the culprit due to its onset and severity.

6) B

This is a typical picture of viral conjunctivitis, which commonly follows upper respiratory tract infections. The discharge tends to be watery and conjunctival hyperaemia may be noted on examination. The most common causative organism is adenovirus serovars 3, 4 and 7, which cause pharyngoconjunctival fever. Adenovirus 8, 19 and 37 cause epidemic keratoconjunctivitis, whereby photophobia is a prominent feature. Coxsackie virus causes acute haemorrhagic conjunctivitis, which is typically found in tropical areas, and conjunctival haemorrhage is marked. HSV can cause follicular conjunctivitis with associated skin vesicles. Molluscum contagiosum may cause conjunctivitis by autoinoculation following the shedding of the virus from skin lesions.

7) A

The lesion being described is a pterygium. Pinguecula and pterygia tend to be more nasal than temporal. The most common cause is ultraviolet (UV) exposure. Unlike pinguecula, a pterygium encroaches on the cornea and invades the Bowman layer. Often, it is painless — patients may complain of dry eyes but it may occasionally become acutely inflamed. Management is often conservative (as for pinguecula) — patients are advised to reduce exposure to UV light and to use regular eye lubricants. Surgical excision is associated with a high recurrence rate.

8) C

The average thickness of the central cornea is between 540 and 560 μm. Generally, a value of below 535 μm is considered thin. Above 565 μm, it is considered thick.

9) D

The layers of the cornea from superficial to deep are:

Epithelium → Bowman layer → Stroma → Descemet membrane → Endothelium

The epithelium is stratified squamous and non-keratinised, compromising of a single layer of columnar basal cells. The Bowman layer is acellular and is formed from collagen fibres. The stroma (substantia propria) makes up the majority of corneal thickness. The Descemet membrane is a basement membrane, which is secreted by the endothelium.

10) D

Bacterial keratitis occurs when ocular defences are compromised (e.g., trauma, contact lens wear and dry eyes). Common pathogens are *Streptococcus* spp., *Staphylococcus aureus* and *Pseudomonas aeruginosa*. Certain bacteria are able to penetrate healthy corneal epithelium such as *Neisseria gonorrhoeae, Neisseria meningitidis, Corynebacterium diphtheriae* and *Haemophilus influenzae*.

11) A

Reduced corneal sensation is a feature of both bacterial and HSV keratitis. In bacterial keratitis, reduced corneal sensation would suggest associated neurotrophic keratopathy. Reduced sensation is more common with HSV. It is rarely associated with microsporidial and fungal keratitis.

12) C

Epithelial keratitis, disciform keratitis and necrotising stromal keratitis may all result from HSV infection. Disciform keratitis is either a hypersensitivity reaction to HSV in the cornea or a result of active infection of the endothelium layer. Gradual blurring of vision, discomfort and redness are common symptoms (discomfort is milder than epithelial disease). Necrotising stromal keratitis causes anterior uveitis with keratic precipitates underlying the area of active stromal infiltration.

13) C

This is a case of herpes zoster ophthalmicus whereby shingles affects the dermatome supplied by the ophthalmic division of the trigeminal nerve. Risk factors for ocular involvement are:

- Age: the signs and symptoms are more severe in the elderly and tend to present most frequently in the 6th and 7th decade
- Immunocompromised (i.e., AIDS)
- Hutchinson sign: this is when there is involvement of the skin on the nose (supplied by the external nasal nerve, a branch of the nasociliary nerve)

14) C

This is a case of congenital syphilis. Systemic signs tend to be sensorineural deafness, a saddle-nose deformity, Hutchinson teeth (small, widely spaced teeth) and sabre tibiae (anterior bowing of the tibia). Ocular features include: anterior uveitis, interstitial keratitis, cataract, optic atrophy, "salt and pepper" retinopathy and the Argyll Robertson pupil. The gradual blurring of vision presenting between the ages of 5–25 years is typical of interstitial keratitis, which involves the corneal stroma.

15) D
Peripheral ulcerative keratitis refers to thinning preferentially affecting the peripheral cornea. Systemic autoimmune diseases result in the upregulation of collagenases. The most common systemic disease associated with this is rheumatoid arthritis. Others include granulomatosis with polyangiitis, polyarteritis nodosa and systemic lupus erythematosus.

16) A
Neurotrophic keratopathy is caused by the failure of re-epithelialisation resulting from corneal anaesthesia. The causes include stroke, tumour, peripheral neuropathy (e.g., from diabetes mellitius) and herpes (simplex and zoster) infections. Bell palsy causes exposure keratopathy.

17) B
Xerophthalmia describes the ocular manifestations that occur in response to vitamin A deficiency. Patients will complain of night blindness, discomfort and loss of vision. Dryness of the conjunctiva manifests with Bitot spots (patches of foamy keratinised epithelium). Dryness of the cornea manifests with lustreless appearance, keratinisation and keratomalacia in severe cases. The WHO's grading of xerophthalmia is:

XN	Night Blindness
X1	Conjunctival xerosis with Bitot spots
X2	Corneal xerosis
X3	Corneal ulceration
XS	Corneal scar
XF	Xerophthalmic fundus

18) B
Filamentary keratopathy is a condition whereby mucus and cellular debris become trapped in a loose area of the corneal epithelium. Patients typically complain of discomfort with a foreign body sensation and occasional photophobia. Filaments can be seen that stain with rose Bengal. Management is aimed at treating the underlying cause. Causes include:

- Excessive contact lens wear
- Neurotrophic keratopathy
- Keratoconjunctivitis sicca
- Surgery: corneal graft, refractive surgery and cataract surgery

19) D
Keratoconus is a disorder where there is progressive thinning of the central corneal stroma with apical protrusion and irregular astigmatism. Most patients do not have a family history. It may be associated with systemic conditions such as Ehlers-Danlos syndrome, Marfan syndrome, osteogenesis imperfecta and Down syndrome. Presentation tends to be with unilateral progressive myopia and astigmatism. LASIK surgery is contraindicated. Patients are advised to avoid eye rubbing, which may exacerbate corneal thinning.

20) B
Fuchs endothelial corneal dystrophy results in a gradual blurring of vision in both eyes, more commonly in females and manifests in middle age. It results in bilateral accelerated endothelial cell loss. Cornea guttata are often present in the early stage; these represent irregular warts excreted by abnormal endothelial cells on Descemet membrane.

21) B
The symptoms this woman exhibits are those of hypercalcaemia ("stones, bones, abdominal moans, and psychic groans"). Ocular manifestations of hypercalcaemia include band keratopathy, which consists of calcium deposition in the epithelial layer, Bowman layer and anterior stroma.

22) D

This young male has Wilson disease, which tends to present with liver disease, basal ganglia dysfunction and psychiatric disturbances as a result of excess deposition of copper. On a slit lamp examination, the Kayser-Fleischer ring may be present, which consists of a brown-yellow zone of copper dusting in the Descemet membrane.

23) D

Some of the contraindications to ocular tissue donation include:
- Death from an unknown cause
- Systemic infections such as HIV, viral hepatitis, syphilis, congenital rubella and tuberculosis
- Prior high-risk behaviour for HIV and hepatitis
- CNS disorders: CJD, dementias, Parkinson disease, multiple sclerosis and motor neurone disease
- Receipt of a transplanted organ
- Haematological malignancy
- Corneal refractive surgery
- Ocular tumours

24) C

Penetrating keratoplasty refers to a surgical procedure that replaces a diseased cornea with a donated, full-thickness corneal graft. Postoperative complications can be subdivided into early and late complications:

Early Complications	Late Complications
- Infection: microbial keratitis, endophthalmitis - Rejection - Wound leak, graft rupture - Raised IOP - Cystoid macular oedema - Fixed dilated pupil (Urrets-Zavalia syndrome)	- Astigmatism - Glaucoma - Late wound dehiscence - Rejection

25) C

This is an anterior necrotising scleritis, which tends to present with gradually worsening pain that radiates to the brow, temple or jaw. It responds poorly to analgesia. There are three main subtypes, according to cause, as outlined in the table below.

Subtype of Anterior Scleritis	Cause and Signs
Vaso-occlusive	• Caused by rheumatoid arthritis • Results in isolated patches of scleral oedema
Granulomatous	• Caused by granulomatosis with polyangiitis and polyarteritis nodosa • Results in diffuse oedema of the sclera, episclera, conjunctiva and adjacent cornea
Surgical	• Usually within 3 weeks of procedure (any type) • Results in a localised necrotising process extending outwards

In this case, the likely cause is the recent trabeculectomy surgery.

Chapter 2 Cataract Questions

1) Epidemiologically, cataracts are:
   A. More prevalent in men than women
   B. Entirely an age-related process
   C. The most common cause of reversible blindness
   D. Not a congenital condition

2) Cataracts are associated with the following systemic diseases:
   A. Marfan syndrome
   B. Osler-Weber-Rendu syndrome
   C. Tuberous sclerosis
   D. Multiple sclerosis

3) Which of the following is **NOT** a symptom arising from the formation of cataracts?
   A. Poor night vision
   B. Reduced contrast sensitivity
   C. Blurred vision for both near and distance
   D. Photophobia

4) Which one of the following types of cataracts is **NOT** age-related?
   A. Nuclear sclerotic
   B. Posterior polar
   C. Cortical
   D. Posterior subcapsular

5) Which of the following is **TRUE** — with age, the lens:
   A. Becomes increasingly curved and has increasing refractive power
   B. Becomes less curved and has decreasing refractive power
   C. Becomes increasingly curved and has decreasing refractive power
   D. Becomes less curved and has increasing refractive power

6) Which of the following is **FALSE** regarding the anatomy of lens?
   A. The lens is biconcave
   B. The lens is avascular
   C. The lens has no neural innervation
   D. The lens is held in place by zonular fibres

7) The contraction of the ciliary muscle ring is related to the shape of the lens via the following mechanism:
   A. Ciliary muscle ring contracts, the ring diameter is reduced and the zonular fibres relax, resulting in the lens becoming rounder
   B. Ciliary muscle ring contracts, the ring diameter is increased and the zonular fibres relax, resulting in the lens becoming rounder
   C. Ciliary muscle ring contracts, the ring diameter is increased and the zonular fibres contract, resulting in the lens becoming flatter
   D. Ciliary muscle ring contracts, the ring diameter is reduced and the zonular fibres relax, resulting in the lens becoming flatter

8) Which of the following is **FALSE** regarding the "pump-leak theory"?
   A. Potassium and amino acids are actively pumped into the anterior portion of the lens via the lens epithelium
   B. All ion movement into the lens is mediated by active transport
   C. Potassium is concentrated in the anterior lens, meanwhile sodium is concentrated in the posterior lens
   D. Intercellular gap junctions facilitate passive diffusion throughout the lens

9) Which of the following is **NOT** a feature of terminal differentiation?
   A. Epithelial cells elongate into lens fibres
   B. There is a loss of cell organelles, including nuclei, ribosomes and mitochondria
   C. The mass of cellular proteins in each cell increases
   D. The cells become less dependent on glycolysis for energy

10) Which of the following refers to a Morgagnian cataract?
    A. A cataract where the lens is completely opacified
    B. A cataract where the lens is partially opacified, but the nucleus has some transparent proteins
    C. Due to the leakage of water from the lens, the cataract has a shrunken anterior capsule
    D. There is cortical liquefaction resulting in the nucleus sinking inferiorly

11) Which one of the following systemic diseases results in the formation of fine, needle-like opacities that resemble a Christmas tree cataract?
    A. Diabetes mellitus
    B. Myotonic dystrophy
    C. Atopic dermatitis
    D. Neurofibromatosis type 2

12) Which one of the following is associated with the formation of snowflake cataracts?
    A. Diabetes mellitus
    B. Neurofibromatosis type 2
    C. Tuberous sclerosis
    D. Von Hippel-Lindau syndrome

13) Which of the following is **FALSE**?
    A. Myopia is associated with the formation of nuclear sclerotic cataract
    B. A nuclear sclerotic cataract can worsen a myopic refractive error
    C. Acute close angle glaucoma can result in subcapsular or capsular opacities
    D. Chronic anterior uveitis is not associated with cataract formation

14) Which of the following drugs is associated with intraoperative floppy iris syndrome?
    A. Atropine
    B. Tamsulosin
    C. Haloperidol
    D. Timolol

15) Which of the following regarding a preoperative ophthalmic assessment is **FALSE**?
   A. A shallow anterior chamber heralds a difficult cataract surgery
   B. Nuclear cataracts tend to require lower ultrasonic energy during phacoemulsification
   C. Ectropion and entropion may increase the likelihood of postoperative endophthalmitis
   D. Trypan blue can be used to overcome a poor red reflex when creating a capsulorrhexis

16) Which of the following is **NOT** an intraocular lens (IOL) power calculation formula?
   A. SRK-T
   B. Hoffer Q
   C. Javal-Schiotz
   D. Holladay 1

17) Which one of the following surgical steps refers to the separation of the lens nucleus and cortex from the capsule?
   A. "Phaco-chop"
   B. "Divide and conquer"
   C. Capsulorrhexis
   D. Hydrodissection

18) Which of the following is **NOT** a sign of posterior lens capsule rupture?
   A. Pupillary dilation and shallowing of anterior chamber
   B. The phaco tip is unable to approach the nucleus as it moves posteriorly
   C. Increased rate of aspiration as vitreous is aspirated by the phaco probe tip
   D. The vitreous gel can be visualised

19) Which of the following perioperative measure is established as the most effective preventative measure for endophthalmitis prophylaxis?
   A. Topical administration of 5% povidone-iodine a few minutes prior to surgery
   B. Topical fluroquinolone in the days leading up to the surgery
   C. Reducing the duration of the surgery
   D. Early suturing of leaking wounds during operation

20) Which of the following is NOT a risk factor for cystoid macular oedema?
   A. Poorly controlled diabetes mellitus
   B. Topical NSAIDs
   C. Posterior capsule rupture
   D. Vitreous loss

21) Which one of the following statements regarding posterior capsular opacification (PCO) is FALSE?
   A. PCO is the most common early complication of cataract surgery
   B. Its causative mechanism involves the proliferation of remnant lens epithelial cells
   C. Capsulorrhexis openings that are in contact with the intraocular lens reduce the incidence of PCO
   D. Epidemiological studies suggest that approximately 50% of all eye patients will eventually develop PCO after cataract surgery

22) Which of the following morphologies is NOT seen in congenital cataract?
   A. Blue dot opacities
   B. Central "oil droplet" opacities
   C. Lamellar opacities
   D. Snowflake opacities

23) A 45-year-old lady presents with a history of increasing difficulty in reading books and newspapers, especially under bright lights. You are told her sole ocular pathology is cataracts. Which one of the following cataract is she MOST likely to have?
   A. Posterior polar
   B. Anterior polar
   C. Nuclear sclerotic
   D. Posterior subscapular

24) Which of the following is NOT a type of congenital cataract?
   A. Zonular
   B. Fusiform
   C. Punctate
   D. Cortical

25) Which of the following is the **MOST** common lens protein?
    A. Alpha crystallin
    B. Beta crystallin
    C. Gamma crystallin
    D. Insoluble albuminoid

Chapter 2

Cataract Answers

1) C

Cataracts may be age-related, congenital or traumatic in their aetiology. They can also be associated with other intraocular diseases. Ionizing radiation and pharmaceutical agents such as steroids can also cause cataracts. There are more common but not exclusive in the elderly. Epidemiological studies point to an increased prevalence among women. It remains the world's leading cause of reversible blindness.

2) A

Cataracts' association with systemic diseases can be categorised by syndrome aetiologies:

Metabolic Disorder	Diabetes, Lowe syndrome, McCune-Albright syndrome, Wilson disease, Fabry disease
Renal Disease	Alport syndrome, Lowe syndrome
Dermatological	Atopic dermatitis, ectodermal dysplasia
Connective Tissue/Skeletal	Myotonic dystrophy, Marfan syndrome, skeletal dysplasia
Central Nervous System	Neurofibromatosis type 2

Although there are literature publications on the association of cataracts and tuberous sclerosis, this is only anecdotal and based on only a few cases series.

3) D

Patients with cataracts may report glare or haloes and streaks surrounding lights and reduced acuity in the presence of bright lights — but this is not photophobia.

Blurred vision, glare, poor night vision, reduced contrast sensitivity and reduced colour sensitivity can be reported symptoms.

4) B

Age-related cataracts are by far the most common cataracts. These can be subdivided by their origin:

Nuclear Sclerotic	Typically causes a myopic shift resulting from the yellowing and hardening of the lens nucleus.
Cortical	Opacification of the lens fibres surrounding the central nucleus with glare being a predominant symptom.
Posterior Subscapular	Opacification of the posterior cortical layer adjacent to the posterior capsule of the lens. Typically seen in younger patients and associated with diabetes and steroid use. Glare is also a predominant symptom.
Posterior Polar	Typically congenital and inherited in an autosomal dominant pattern. They project forward from the centre of the posterior capsule to penetrate the lens cortex.

5) A

The ageing lens becomes increasing curved with time, resulting in an increase in its refractive power.

6) A

The lens is a biconvex structure that is avascular and non-innervated. It is held in place by zonular fibres that arise from the ciliary body and attach to the equatorial region of the lens. The lens is suspended posteriorly to the iris. It divides the eye into posterior and anterior segments. It is comprised of three layers that include, from central to peripheral, the nucleus, cortex and capsule.

7) A

The ciliary muscle is a ring that is attached to the lens by zonular fibres. Upon contraction, the diameter of the ring counterintuitively reduces. Therefore the zonular fibres are relaxed and the tension force on the lens is also reduced, resulting in the lens becoming rounder.

Given this, the ciliary muscles play an important role in accommodation and adjusting the focusing of the light reflecting from the objects to land on the fovea. Contraction is mediated by the parasympathetic activation of M3 muscarinic receptors.

8) B

The "pump-leak" theory refers to the combination of active and passive transport of ions in and out of the lens. The theory stipulates that potassium and other molecules are pumped into the lens via ATPase and exchange pumps located in the epithelium of the lens anteriorly. These then diffuse to the posterior lens via passive diffusion and leave the lens due to membrane permeability in the back of the lens.

Conversely, sodium passively flows in through the posterior lens down the concentration and electrochemical gradient and is actively exchanged with potassium in the anterior lens via Na^+/K^+-ATPase exchangers.

9) D

Terminal differentiation refers to the process by which the lens epithelial cells lose their organelles and elongate into lens fibres. There is an increase in the intracellular protein mass, even as these cells lose their organelles. In doing so, they form a homogenous cytoplasm that is optically advantageous.

However, in losing their mitochondria, the cells switch from oxidative phosphorylation and increasingly rely on glycolysis, the hexose monophosphotase shunt and aldose reductase pathway for energy.

10) D

Cataract maturity can be classified as:

Immature	There are still some transparent proteins and the lens is only partially opaque.
Mature	All of the proteins in the lens are now opaque.
Hypermature	There is a leakage of water from the lens resulting in a shrunken, withered appearance of the anterior capsule.
Morgagnian	A type of hypermature cataract where there is liquefaction of the cortex and subsequent settlement of the nucleus inferiorly.

11) B

Patients with myotonic dystrophy typically present with cortical opacities that tend to resemble a Christmas tree cataract due to their iridescence and fine, needle-like morphology. This is seen in almost 90% of patients with myotonic dystrophy and typically presents at the age of 30–40 years.

With time, these fine opacities develop into wedge-shaped cortical and sometimes subcapsular cataracts. In this phase, they are often likened to a star shape.

12) A

Patient with poorly controlled diabetes may have a hyperglycaemic aqueous humour, which results in a diffusion of glucose into the lens. Its subsequent metabolisation and accumulation in the form of sorbitol result in an increased oncotic pressure, driving water into the lens.

This can lead to limited and temporary change in the shape of the lens and its refractory index, which fluctuates with the corresponding rise or fall in plasma glucose levels. It can also, albeit rarely, cause the formation of snowflake cataracts in young patients. These are pathognomonic of diabetes. Incidentally, age-related cataract formation takes place from an earlier age in patients with diabetes.

13) D

Chronic anterior uveitis remains one of the most common causes of secondary cataracts. There is a close association with the degree and duration of inflammation. Unfortunately, the use of topical steroids, whilst indicated as treatment, may exacerbate cataract formation.

High-grade myopia is associated with the formation of posterior capsular and nuclear sclerosis cataracts, both of which can induce or exacerbate a myopic refractive error.

14) B

The intraoperative floppy iris syndrome (IFIS) refers to a triad of:

- A "floppy" iris that transverses the incision site
- Iris prolapse
- Pupillary constriction during the operation

Tamsulosin increases the risk of IFIS, although suspending it preoperatively has not been shown to be effective in reducing IFIS. Newer generations of antipsychotic medications such as risperidone can also increase the risk of IFIS.

15) B

In creating a capsulorrhexis, the operating surgeon creates an opening in the anterior capsule, allowing them access to the cortex and nucleus. A poor red reflex can make it difficult for capsulorrhexis creation, but this can be overcome to good effect by using Trypan blue.

With a shallow anterior chamber, performing a capsulorrhexis is difficult due to poor manoeuvrability and the lack of flattening of the anterior lens capsule.

Nuclear cataracts tend to be harder than cortical or posterior subcapsular cataracts. Hence, higher phacoemulsification energy may be required.

Ectropion and entropion may increase the likelihood of postoperative endophthalmitis, as can chronic conjunctivitis, dacryocystitis, blepharitis and tear film abnormalities.

16) C

Postoperative refractive outcomes are predetermined using biometry and power calculation to determine the desired intraocular lenses power. Many such formulae exist and common examples include SRK-T, Haigis and Holladay 1 and 2. Some are used more than others in certain situations (e.g., Hoffer Q for those with very short eyes).

17) D

Hydrodissection refers to the injection of fluid via a blunt cannula to separate the lens cortex and nucleus from the capsule. Meanwhile, "divide and conquer" and "phaco-chop" both refer to lens disassembly techniques in which the nucleus is emulsified and aspirated.

As stated above, capsulorrhexis refers to the opening in the anterior capsule, allowing access to the cortex and nucleus.

18) C

Rupture of the posterior lens capsule can result in vitreous loss and downward movement of the lens into the vitreous chamber. Intraoperative signs of this include:

- The sudden deepening of the anterior chamber and pupil dilation
- The nucleus will move posteriorly as the phaco tip approaches it

- As vitreous is aspirated into the tip, there may be a noticeable drop in aspiration
- The vitreous may come in the line of sight

Poorly managed posterior capsular rupture can result in retinal detachment, cystoid macular oedema, glaucoma and uveitis.

19) A
Whilst (A), (C) and (D) are all correct, instillation of povidone-iodine 5% onto the ocular surface at least 3–5 minutes prior to surgery is recommended and has the highest quality evidence to support its efficacy. Preoperative antibiotic prophylaxis is given in some centres across the world, however, the evidence of its efficacy is lacking.

20) B
Cystoid macular oedema (CMO) remains one of the most common causes of postoperative visual loss. Peri- and postoperative release of inflammatory mediators results in increased permeability in the foveal capillaries resulting in CMO.

Topical NSAIDs can reduce postoperative inflammation and have been shown to be efficacious in reducing the incidence of CMO. Meanwhile, poorly controlled diabetes, vitreous loss and posterior capsule rupture are associated with an increased risk of CMO.

21) A
PCO is one of the most common late complications of cataract surgery. Studies show that almost half of all patients will eventually develop PCO. Symptoms typically include a gradual blurring of vision and glare. In patients who have significant visual symptoms, a capsulotomy may be indicated where an opening is created in the posterior capsule. PCO is thought to be caused by the proliferation of epithelial cells that were left behind during cataract surgery.

22) D
Snowflake opacities are seen in young diabetic patients, albeit rarely, and can be self-resolving. Blue dot opacities are common and innocuous as congenital opacities. Central "oil droplet" opacities are associated with galactosaemia.

Lamellar opacities occur anteriorly and posteriorly in the lamella region of the lens and can have radial extensions. These can be hereditary, portraying an autosomal dominant inheritance pattern, in association with certain metabolic disorders and can also be associated with intrauterine infection during pregnancy.

23) D

Posterior subscapular cataracts often result in difficulty with near vision and glare. They can be rapidly progressive and are often seen in a younger demographic compared to nuclear sclerotic or cortical cataracts. Risk factors include steroid use, diabetes, uveitis and radiation.

Nuclear sclerotic cataract may affect distance vision as opposed to near vision due to a myopic shift. A progressive loss of vision from anterior polar cataracts would not often be seen at someone of this age. Posterior polar cataracts are typically congenital, displaying an autosomal dominant pattern of inheritance. However, given their rarity, they are not very well characterised.

24) D

A cortical cataract is an age-related cataract.

Zonular cataracts account for almost 50% of all congenital cataracts that are visually significant. They usually affect both eyes with the opacity usually showing a sharp demarcation. They tend to form just before or shortly after birth.

Fusiform cataracts are spindle-shaped opacities. There is a strong genetic disposition, and they can often resemble a coral in their morphology and hence are often also referred to as coralliform.

Punctate cataracts are also known as blue dot cataracts and are the most common type of congenital cataracts. The vast majority do not have any impact on vision.

25) B

Eighty to 90 percent of soluble proteins in the lens are crystallins. The most common of which is beta (51%), followed by alpha (31%) and gamma (2%). With age, the concentration of both soluble and non-soluble proteins increases. This results in light scattering and contributes to the formation of cataracts.

Chapter 3

Glaucoma Questions

1) According to epidemiological studies, glaucoma accounts for approximately what percentage of blindness worldwide?
   A. 1%
   B. 30%
   C. 3%
   D. 10%

2) A 57-year-old lady with a history of diabetes and primary open angle glaucoma (POAG) presents to her optometrist with worsening visual field defects. She is also myopic. Which of the following is **NOT** a known risk factor for POAG?
   A. Increased intraocular pressure (IOP)
   B. Myopia
   C. Diabetes
   D. Female gender

3) Which of these statements regarding the ciliary body is **FALSE**?
   A. The ciliary muscle is innervated by the parasympathetic branch of the oculomotor nerve
   B. The pars plicata is anterior to the pars plana
   C. The pigmented epithelium is involved in active fluid transport using Na^+/K^+-ATPase pumps
   D. The ciliary body produces aqueous fluid at a rate of around 2–3 $\mu L/min$

4) Which of the following statements about aqueous humour is **FALSE**?
   A. It is produced at a rate of approximately 2–3 µL/min
   B. It has an estimated turnover rate of around 1.0–1.5% of the anterior chamber volume per minute
   C. Aqueous humour contains approximately the same protein concentration as plasma
   D. Its concentration of glucose is around 75% of plasma glucose concentration

5) Select the correct order (anterior to posterior) in which structures appear on gonioscopy.
   A. Schwalbe line, non-pigmented trabecular meshwork, pigmented trabecular meshwork, scleral spur, ciliary body, iris processes
   B. Schwalbe line, pigmented trabecular meshwork, non-pigmented trabecular meshwork, scleral spur, ciliary body, iris processes
   C. Schwalbe line, non-pigmented trabecular meshwork, pigmented trabecular meshwork, ciliary body, scleral spur, iris processes
   D. Non-pigmented trabecular meshwork, Schwalbe line, pigmented trabecular meshwork, scleral spur, ciliary body, iris processes

6) Schwalbe line is:
   A. A projection from the inner aspect of the anterior sclera
   B. A line that represents the termination of Descemet membrane
   C. The most posteriorly observed structure via gonioscopy
   D. A transition from the ciliary body to the retina

7) Aqueous humour passes through the trabecular meshwork (TM) as it exits the eye. Which of these statements regarding the TM is **FALSE**?
   A. The TM accounts for 90% of the aqueous outflow
   B. Pigmentation of the TM varies from pale-tan to dark brown, with the anterior aspect being darker pigmented
   C. It is divided into the three anatomical sections known as the uveal, corneoscleral and juxtacanalicular TM
   D. Aqueous outflow from the Schlemm canal drains into the episcleral veins

8) Anterior chamber depth:
   A. Is lower in women than in men
   B. Decreases with age
   C. Is decreased in extreme myopia
   D. Is not associated with anterior chamber volume

9) Primary glaucoma is not associated with an underlying eye pathology. Which of the following statements regarding primary open angle glaucoma (POAG) and primary angle closure glaucoma (PACG) is **TRUE**?
   A. Optineurin and myocilin genes have been identified as contributory to the pathogenesis of PACG
   B. Myopia is associated with PACG whereas hypermetropia is associated with POAG
   C. History of vascular disease such as stroke or ischaemic heart disease increases the risk of POAG
   D. POAG more commonly affects females than men

10) A 68-year-old Afro-Caribbean man is seen for the first time in the glaucoma clinic. On examination, he appears to have white foci of necrosis in the superficial aspect of the lens, with an irregular pupil. What is the likely diagnosis?
    A. Acute primary angle closure (APAC)
    B. Normal tension glaucoma
    C. Late stages of a resolved APAC
    D. Posner-Schlossman syndrome

11) A 60-year-old man presents to the A&E department with intense periocular pain and acute unilateral visual loss in his right eye, which is red. A diagnosis of acute primary angle closure (APAC) is made. The patient has just returned from a cruise holiday, having used motion sickness patches to prevent sea sickness. Since his return, he has spent his days watching television in a bright room while in a supine position. He complains of being in a lot of emotional stress with his current housing situation. Which of the following is likely to have been a precipitating factor?
   A. A tropical disease from his travels
   B. Watching television in a bright room
   C. Supine position
   D. Motion sickness patches

12) Which of the following histological changes is **NOT** seen in glaucoma?
   A. Loss of the outer nuclear layer of the retina
   B. Posterior bowing of the lamina cribrosa
   C. Loss of ganglion cells in the retina
   D. Peripapillary atrophy

13) A patient has been seen by her optometrist and referred to the glaucoma clinic. Which of the following investigation results is suggestive of glaucoma?
   A. A cup:disc ratio of 0.3 in the right eye and 0.45 in the left eye
   B. A cup:disc ratio of 0.26 in the left eye
   C. Diffuse loss of the neuro-retinal rim and a saucerised disc, visualised with a slit-lamp
   D. Central corneal thickness (CCT) of 540 microns

14) Goldmann applanation tonometry (GAT) is used to measure intraocular pressure (IOP). Select the most appropriate statement regarding GAT.
   A. The Robert-Sacks principle is used to approximate IOP
   B. A flattened area of 5.07 mm during tonometry enables accurate IOP measurements
   C. The formula $P = F/A$ is used to calculate the pressure (P), whereby F is the force applied by the device to flatten the area (A) of the cornea
   D. GAT provides an exact value of IOP

15) Drugs that decrease aqueous production are commonly used in the management of glaucoma. What is the mechanism of action of beta-blockers?
   A. Reduces adenylyl cyclase activity, which in turn decreases active fluid transport using Na^+/K^+-ATPase pumps
   B. Blocks enzyme production of bicarbonate ions
   C. Increases uveoscleral outflow
   D. Stimulates sphincter pupillae contraction

16) A 62-year-old man is using topical latanoprost as a first-line treatment for his glaucoma. What is thought to be the principal mechanism of action of prostaglandin analogues in glaucoma treatment?
   A. Increases trabecular outflow
   B. Increases uveoscleral outflow
   C. Decreases aqueous production
   D. Creates an osmotic gradient to encourage movement of water from vitreous to blood stream

17) A 52-year-old woman receives eye drops to treat her glaucoma. She presents to her GP with increasing redness in her eyes. Which drug is the most likely culprit?
   A. An allergic reaction to medication
   B. Topical timolol
   C. Topical bimatoprost
   D. Topical apraclonidine

18) A 49-year-old woman with a history of glaucoma attends the glaucoma clinic. After taking a full history, you note that she is allergic to sulfonamides. Which of the following medications would you avoid in this patient?
   A. Brimonidine
   B. Timolol
   C. Pilocarpine
   D. Acetazolamide

19) Which of the following statements regarding pilocarpine is **FALSE**?
    A. It can cause narrowing of the anterior chamber by relaxing tension of the zonular fibres
    B. It is a direct cholinergic agonist
    C. It inhibits acetylcholinesterase
    D. It increases aqueous flow, thus reducing IOP

20) A patient complains of a bitter taste after using his eye drops. He has a past medical history of glaucoma and is noted to be taking an anti-glaucoma medication. Which medication is likely to be responsible for his current presentation?
    A. Latanoprost
    B. Bimatoprost
    C. Dorzolamide
    D. Pilocarpine

21) Which of the following is an indication for a trabeculectomy?
    A. A previously failed trabeculectomy
    B. Neovascular glaucoma
    C. Conjunctival scarring
    D. Elevated IOP despite optimisation of medical therapies

22) Which of the following is **NOT** associated with pseudoexfoliation syndrome?
    A. Wider variations in IOP
    B. Deeper anterior chamber angle
    C. Spontaneous lens dislocation
    D. Earlier cataract formation

23) A 78-year-old man presents to an outpatient clinic with reduced vision in his right eye, associated with sudden onset pain and conjunctival hyperaemia. His IOP is measured at 45 mmHg. On examination, the cornea is of a foggy appearance without any keratic precipitate. He has a hypermature cataract and an open anterior chamber angle. Which of the following is the most likely diagnosis?
    A. Phacolytic glaucoma
    B. Phacoantigenic glaucoma
    C. Iridocorneal endothelial syndrome
    D. Fuchs heterochromic iridocyclitis

24) Sturge-Weber syndrome:
   A. Always affects both eyes and commonly results in a bilateral glaucoma
   B. Is a congenital neuro-oculocutaneous syndrome
   C. Rarely results in ocular conjunctival and choroidal haemangiomas
   D. Is not associated with buphthalmos or anisometropia

25) In which secondary angle closure glaucoma does peripheral anterior synechiae (PAS) extend anterior to the Schwalbe line?
   A. Iridocorneal endothelial syndrome
   B. Fuchs heterochromic iridocyclitis
   C. Neovascular glaucoma
   D. Axenfeld-Rieger syndrome

Chapter 3 Glaucoma Answers

1) D
Glaucoma accounts for around 10% of global blindness. In 2040, the worldwide prevalence of glaucoma will be an estimated 112 million people. It is currently the leading cause of irreversible blindness and the third leading cause of global blindness after cataract (35%) and uncorrected refractive error (20%).

2) D
Risk factors for POAG include increasing age, raised IOP (A), Afro-Caribbean ethnicity (tends to present with more severe and younger onset, and with more resistance to treatment), family history (history of 1st degree relative poses a 1 in 8 risk), diabetes (C), hypertension and refractive abnormalities such as myopia (B). Female gender (D) is not a known risk factor for POAG (but rather primary angle closure glaucoma).

3) C
(C) is incorrect, as it is the non-pigmented epithelial cells that contain Na^+/K^+-ATPase pumps and are involved in the production of aqueous humour. The anterior portion of the ciliary body is called the pars plicata (B), consisting of the ciliary muscle and ciliary processes. The posterior 4 mm is referred to as the pars plana. The ciliary epithelium is formed of two layers: the pigmented epithelium, which is continuous with the retinal-pigmented epithelium and adjacent to the stroma, and the non-pigmented epithelium, which is continuous with the retina and adjacent to the aqueous humour. The major innervation to the ciliary muscle is the parasympathetic branch of the oculomotor nerve (CN III). The ciliary body produces aqueous fluid at a rate of 2–3 microlitres per minute (D).

4) C
The protein concentration in aqueous humour is less than 1% of the plasma protein concentration. This equates to around 5–16 mg/100 ml of protein within aqueous.

5) A

Gonioscopy is used in conjunction with slit lamps in order to visualise the iridocorneal angle. The correct order (from posterior to anterior) of structures can be remembered using the mnemonic "I Can See Till Schwalbe line", which translates to **I**ris processes, **C**iliary body, **S**cleral spur, **T**rabecular meshwork and **S**chwalbe line. This means (A) is correct, as the most anterior structure is Schwalbe line and the most posterior structure being the iris processes. The non-pigmented trabecular meshwork is anterior to the pigmented trabecular meshwork.

6) B

Schwalbe line demarcates the most peripheral termination of Descemet membrane. It is the most anterior structure of the angle, not the most posterior (C). The line appears as a white-yellow line. It is the scleral spur that is a fibrous wedge-shaped projection extending from the inner part of the anterior sclera (A).

7) B

(B) is incorrect as the pigmented TM is located posteriorly to the non-pigmented TM. Ninety per cent of the aqueous outflow is via the TM (A), whereas the remaining 10% flows via the uveoscleral pathway and the iris.

8) B

Anterior chamber depth decreases with age.

9) C

POAG is associated with the optineurin and myocilin genes (A). (B) is incorrect as POAG is associated with myopia and PACG with hypermetropia. Vascular disease is known to increase the risk of POAG (C). POAG is more common in males than females (D).

10) C

This question is alluding to some of the features observed in resolved APAC (C). The white foci of necrosis in the lens describe glaucomflecken. Iris atrophy with spiral-like configurations, cataracts, irregular pupils and glaucomflecken may be observed in the late stages of a resolved APAC.

11) D
Motion sickness patches (D) have a mydriatic effect that can precipitate an episode of APAC. If he had contracted a form of tropical disease (A), he would likely have more systemic symptoms. Sitting in a bright room (B) may in fact alleviate some of his symptoms by inducing miosis. A typical history of spending time in a dark environment is commonly associated with APAC. A semi-prone position is a more likely precipitating factor than a supine position (C).

12) A
Glaucoma principally involves the loss of retinal ganglion cells and their axons (C). There is no loss of the outer nuclear layer (A).

13) C
Glaucoma is investigated using various modalities including, but not limited to, tonometry, pachymetry, gonioscopy, a slit lamp examination, perimetry and optical coherence tomography (OCT). Tonometry is used to measure intraoculare pressure (IOP). Pachymetry measures corneal thickness. A normal CCT is 540 microns (D). CCT affects IOP measurements. Gonioscopy measures angle width; a Grade 0 angle on gonioscopy is suggestive of an angle-closure glaucoma. A slit lamp examination is used to visualise cup:disc ratios; a normal cup:disc ratio is 0.3 or less. A disparity in the cup:disc ratio between the two eyes of ≥0.2 is suspicious of glaucoma. A slit lamp examination also enables visualisation of the optic disc, whereby thinning of the neuro-retinal rim (NRR) and enlarged optic disc is suggestive of glaucoma.

14) C
The Imbert-Fick principle is applied for dry, thin-walled spheres to measure the pressure within the sphere. It is used in GAT to approximate the IOP. The formula used is: Pressure inside sphere (P) = Force needed to flatten surface of sphere (F) / area of flattening (A). Force is varied to achieve an area of flattening of 3.06 mm in order to derive the pressure.

15) A
Beta-blockers inhibit activity of beta-adrenergic receptors 1 and 2, which stimulate cAMP production by adenylyl cyclase, and hence active fluid transport using Na^+/K^+-ATPase pumps (A). Carbonic anhydrase

inhibitors block enzyme production of bicarbonate ions (B). The uveoscleral flow (C) is increased by drugs such as prostaglandins and alpha-2 agonists. Miotics and parasympathomimetics like pilocarpine and carbachol stimulate sphincter pupillae contraction.

16) B
Prostaglandin analogues such as latanoprost and bimatoprost work by increasing the uveoscleral outflow (B). The trabecular outflow is increased (A) by miotics, such as pilocarpine, through the action of ciliary muscle contraction.

17) C
Prostaglandin analogues like bimatoprost (C) are commonly used as first-line treatment for glaucoma as they are the most effective treatment in lowering the IOP in POAG. However, the most commonly associated side effect is conjunctival hyperaemia. Latanoprost is associated with a milder side-effect profile compared with bimatoprost, a prostaglandin analogue with a greater IOP-lowering effect.

18) D
The use of acetazolamide (D) in patients with sulfonamide allergies is contraindicated due to the risk of cross-reactivity.

19) C
Pilocarpine is a direct cholinergic agonist (B), and therefore does not act indirectly by inhibiting acetylcholinesterase (C). Pilocarpine is used in the treatment of glaucoma, and its mode of action involves increasing drainage of aqueous fluid through the trabecular meshwork.

20) C
Dorzolamide, a topical carbonic anhydrase inhibitor, is known to cause stinging and a transient bitter taste following administration.

21) D
Trabeculectomy is preferred in the surgical management of glaucoma if medical management has not been sufficient (D). The other indications in the question relate to indications for aqueous shunting, where there is a poor prognosis for successful trabeculectomy surgery (e.g., uveitis, neovascular glaucoma, conjunctival scarring).

22) B

Pseudoexfoliation syndrome is a disease in which there is abnormal deposition of fibrillar extracellular material in the anterior chamber, including the trabecular meshwork. Patients tend to have narrower anterior chamber angles. Secondary glaucomas such as pseudoexfoliation syndrome are associated with increased variation in the IOP compared with primary glaucomas (A). Studies have shown a causal relationship between pseudoexfoliation syndrome and the earlier formation of cataracts (D).

23) A

The presentation described in the question is typical of phacolytic glaucoma (A). As the name suggests, phacolytic glaucoma is caused by the leaking of a mature or hypermature cataract. Removal of the cataracts cures the glaucoma. Due to the lack of keratic precipitate, phacoantigenic glaucoma (B) and Fuchs heterochromic iridocyclitis (D) are unlikely. Iridocorneal endothelial syndrome (ICE) tends to occur in younger patients.

24) B

Sturge-Weber syndrome, also known as encephalotrigeminal angiomatosis, is a congenital syndrome with neurological, ocular and cutaneous manifestations (B). The ocular manifestations of Sturge-Weber syndrome result from haemangiomas of the conjunctiva, episclera and choroid (C). It can result in glaucoma, which is present in 30–70% of patients with Sturge-Weber syndrome, and is often ipsilateral to the side of the port wine stain, but can sometimes, but not always, manifest bilaterally (A). It is also associated with buphthalmos, anisometropia and amblyopia.

25) A

In iridocorneal endothelial (ICE) syndrome, abnormal corneal endothelium migrates posteriorly beyond Schwalbe line (A). On gonioscopy, the peripheral anterior synechiae may be seen extending above Schwalbe line.

Chapter 4
Medical Retina and Vitreoretinal Surgery Questions

1) Which one of the following statements regarding the anatomy of the retina is **FALSE**?
   A. The clinical macula corresponds to the anatomical fovea
   B. The clinical macula is around 5.5 mm in diameter
   C. The optic disc is around 1.5 mm in diameter
   D. The anatomical macula refers to the area of the retina, which has two or more layers of ganglion cells

2) During embryogenesis, which structure originates from the neuroectoderm?
   A. Iris
   B. Sclera
   C. Vitreous
   D. Cornea

3) Which of the comparisons between direct and indirect ophthalmoscopy is **FALSE**?
   A. Direct ophthalmoscopy provides a higher magnification than indirect ophthalmoscopy
   B. The image observed with direct ophthalmoscopy is real and inverted, unlike indirect ophthalmoscopy, through which virtual and erect images are seen
   C. Direct ophthalmoscopy has a smaller field of view
   D. Direct ophthalmoscopes are monocular instruments whereas indirect ophthalmoscopes provide a binocular view

4) Hypofluorescence on fundus fluorescein angiography is suggestive of which of the following diseases?
   A. Central retinal artery occlusion
   B. Drusen in age-related macular degeneration
   C. Retinal pigment epithelium (RPE) defect
   D. Retinal detachment

5) What are cotton wool spots?
   A. Swollen axons caused by ischaemia
   B. Discrete deposits of protein-rich material, giving them a yellow appearance
   C. Retinal oedema
   D. Microaneurysms

6) What is the mechanism of action of panretinal photocoagulation (PRP)?
   A. Reduces intraocular oxygen requirement, hence increasing production of endogenous anti-vascular endothelial growth factor (VEGF)
   B. Reduces intraocular oxygen requirement, hence decreasing the production of VEGF
   C. Damages the peripheral retina to increase the hypoxic drive
   D. Stimulates healing of the retina

7) A 75-year-old man with a history of poorly controlled type 2 diabetes describes a recent onset of blurred vision with the appearance of floaters and flashes of light. Which of the following treatment options would be most suitable in managing this complication of diabetic retinopathy?
   A. Panretinal photocoagulation
   B. Phacoemulsification
   C. Trabeculectomy
   D. Vitrectomy and delamination

8) Which of the following retinal changes is observed in Grade 2 hypertensive retinopathy?
   A. Minimal arteriolar narrowing only
   B. Retinal hemorrhage and hard exudates
   C. Arteriovenous nipping
   D. Papilloedema

9) Which of the following is least likely to be a complication of retinal vein occlusion?
   A. Rubeosis iridis
   B. Macular oedema
   C. Retinal neovascularisation
   D. Macular hole

10) Which of the following investigations should be considered after a diagnosis of retinal artery occlusion is made?
    A. Carotid duplex scan
    B. Transoesophageal echocardiogram
    C. Transthoracic echocardiogram
    D. B-scan ultrasound

11) A 65-year-old man presents with reduced visual acuity of his left eye. The OCT scan shows changes consistent with cystoid macular oedema. Which of the following is a risk factor for his condition?
    A. UV light exposure
    B. Raised intraocular pressure
    C. Retinitis pigmentosa
    D. Macular degeneration seen in Fuchs dystrophy

12) A 75-year-old woman complains of a unilateral loss of central vision and spared peripheral vision. She has no significant past medical history. A procedure involving a vitrectomy and the use of gas tamponade resulted in an improvement of her vision. Which of the following conditions is the most likely cause of her initial central vision loss?
    A. Age-related macular degeneration
    B. Macular hole
    C. Central serous chorioretinopathy
    D. Cystoid macular oedema

13) A stressed out 35-year-old man complains of a grey spot in the centre of his vision unilaterally. On a slit lamp examination, a dome-shaped elevation is seen at the fovea. Fluorescein angiography confirms the diagnosis. What is the most likely diagnosis?
    A. Age-related macular degeneration
    B. Central serous chorioretinopathy
    C. Cystoid macular oedema
    D. Macular hole

14) An 85-year-old female, who was previously experiencing progressive bilateral central loss of vision and distortion of straight lines, now develops marked central visual loss. Which of the following features is least likely to be associated with the disorder described?
   A. Choroidal neovascularisation
   B. Drusen lesions
   C. RPE atrophy
   D. Operculum

15) A tall, slender man with scoliosis complains of an enlarging dark shadow obstructing the right side of his vision, along with seeing flashes of light. He has no other significant comorbidities. Which type of retinal detachment is this man most likely suffering from?
   A. Rhegmatogenous retinal detachment
   B. Tractional retinal detachment
   C. Exudative retinal detachment
   D. Posterior vitreous detachment

16) Which of the following is caused by degeneration of the peripheral retina, typically with splitting between the inner nuclear and outer plexiform layers of the retina? It is present more commonly in hypermetropes.
   A. Tractional retinal detachment
   B. Serous retinal detachment
   C. Acquired retinoschisis
   D. Rhegmatogenous retinal detachment

17) In retinal detachment, between which structures does fluid accumulate?
   A. The outer plexiform layer and outer nuclear layer
   B. The inner nuclear layer and outer plexiform layer
   C. The ganglion cell layer and inner plexiform layer
   D. The retinal pigment epithelium and photoreceptor layer

18) During a routine check-up of an 18-month-old child, a GP notes macular lesions on fundoscopy. The lesions are round and sharply demarcated, consistent with vitelliform lesions. Given the features on fundoscopy, which of the following is the most likely diagnosis?
    A. Best disease
    B. Juvenile retinoschisis
    C. Stargardt disease
    D. Cone-rod dystrophy

19) A 2-year-old presents with poor vision. On examination, leukocoria is noted. His newborn screening check was normal. Which is the most likely culpable gene?
    A. 13q14
    B. 11q13
    C. ABCA4
    D. OCA1

20) A 57-year-old lady has a rare autoimmune disease causing floaters and painless blurred vision. On fundoscopy, some cream-coloured ovoid patches are noted. She is HLA-A29 positive. What is the likely diagnosis?
    A. Birdshot chorioretinopathy
    B. Acute retinal necrosis
    C. Progressive outer retinal necrosis
    D. Juvenile idiopathic arthritis

21) A 14-year-old boy presents with unilateral ptosis, which has gradually progressed to bilateral ptosis. His mother has noticed that he has difficulty hearing and loses his balance easily. Which of the following investigations would be useful in aiding the diagnosis?
    A. PCR
    B. Rubella antigen detection by monoclonal antibody
    C. Fundus fluorescein angiography
    D. ECG

22) An immunocompetent 68-year-old man presents with acute vision loss in one eye, along with floaters and flashes. A physical examination revealed some anterior uveitis and patchy retinal opacification. His diagnosis is confirmed with PCR. Which organism is likely to have caused the condition described?
    A. Herpes simplex virus (HSV)
    B. Cytomegalovirus (CMV)
    C. Varicella zoster virus (VZV)
    D. Rubella virus

23) A 28-year-old lady presents with blurred vision and floaters. On fundoscopy, a pigmented scar and a nearby satellite lesion is seen. Which of the following is the most appropriate treatment option?
    A. Systemic prednisolone, pyrimethamine and sulfadiazine
    B. Intravitreal ganciclovir
    C. Intravitreal foscarnet
    D. Systemic flucytosine

24) A 34-year-old man with a previous hospital admission with *Pneumocystis* pneumonia presents to his GP with dense white confluent retinal opacifications and retinal haemorrhages, described as a "pizza pie" appearance. What is the most likely diagnosis?
    A. Toxoplasma retinitis
    B. CMV retinitis
    C. Congenital rubella
    D. Sarcoidosis

25) A 38-year-old man presents with a central loss of vision. He is noted to have bilaterally reduced visual acuity and colour vision. He is particularly unable to distinguish between green and red. He has a past medical history of hypertension, recent myocardial infarction, atrial fibrillation, alcohol excess and treated tuberculosis. Which of his medications is the most likely culprit for his current presentation?
    A. Ethambutol
    B. Amiodarone
    C. Alcohol
    D. Linezolid

Chapter 4
Medical Retina and Vitreoretinal Surgery Answers

1) B
It is the *anatomical* macula that has a diameter of around 5.5 mm (B). The macula is centrally located in the retina, and is responsible for central, high resolution coloured vision. The anatomical macula is histologically defined as having two or more layers of ganglion cells (D). The clinical macula, which is around 1.5 mm in diameter, is synonymous with the anatomical fovea (A). The fovea is further subdivided into the foveal avascular zone, foveola and umbo.

2) A
The epithelial lining of the iris (A) and ciliary body, along with the retina and optic nerve derive from the neuroectoderm. The surface ectoderm develops into the lens, corneal epithelium and eyelids. The neural crest cells develop into the corneal stroma and endothelium whereas the mesoderm develops into the sclera (B), blood vessels, and vitreous (C).

3) B
Direct ophthalmoscopes are monocular instruments (D), which have a higher magnification (A) but smaller field of view (C), compared with indirect ophthalmoscopes. Images observed through direct ophthalmoscopes are real and erect, whereas images from indirect ophthalmoscopes are virtual and inverted.

4) A
Fluorescein angiography allows visualisation of choroidal and retinal vasculature. An area of vascular filling defect, as seen in a central retinal artery occlusion (A) can cause hypofluorescence. RPE defects (C) are hyperfluorescent due to a window defect. Autofluorescence can occur with drusen (B).

5) A
Cotton wool spots represent damage to the nerve fibre layer caused by microinfarctions. It is one of the clinical features of diabetic retinopathy. Other features in diabetes retinopathy include hard exudates (B), retinal oedema (C), microaneurysms (D) and dot/blot haemorrhages.

6) B
Panretinal photocoagulation (PRP) damages and sacrifices the peripheral retina, reducing the oxygen requirement of the retina, and hence decreasing VEGF production. This helps to attenuate the process of neovascularisation.

7) D
The blurred vision, floaters and flashes (photopsia) are suggestive of a retinal detachment. Fibrovascular proliferation in diabetic retinopathy can lead to tractional retinal detachment. It is managed with vitrectomy and delamination (D). Other complications of diabetic retinopathy include diabetic maculopathy, vitreous haemorrhage, rubeosis iridis, cataract and ocular motor nerve palsies.

8) C
Compression of the veins at arteriovenous crossings, termed arteriovenous nipping, along with arteriolar narrowing is seen in a Grade 2 disease. Minimal arteriolar narrowing (A) is seen in a Grade 1 disease. Copper wiring, cotton wool exudates and hard exudates (C) are observed in a Grade 3 disease. A Grade 4 disease is defined by the presence of papilloedema.

9) D
The main complications associated with retinal vein occlusion include macular oedema (B) and neovascularisation of the retina (C) and the iris (rubeosis iridis) (A). A macular hole (D) is not a known complication of retinal vein occlusion. Rubeosis iridis can lead to neovascular glaucoma.

10) A
The most common cause of arterial occlusion is embolisation, frequently originating from the carotid artery. Carotid duplex scans are used to assess the severity of carotid artery disease.

Medical Retina and Vitreoretinal Surgery Answers

11) C

Cystoid macular oedema occurs when fluid within the retina coalesces into cystic-like spaces. The causes of cystoid macular oedema include diabetic maculopathy, retinitis pigmentosa, retinal vein occlusion, Irvine-Gass syndrome, pars planitis, adrenaline, niacin and E2-prostaglandin.

12) B

Macular disorders typically impair central vision, whilst leaving the peripheral vision intact. Macular hole (B) is an age-related idiopathic loss of neural tissue at the fovea. It may resolve spontaneously. Surgical removal of the vitreous (vitrectomy) and closure of the macular hole with gas tamponade can be used to improve vision. Although age-related macular degeneration (AMD) (A) is associated with increasing age, it tends to occur bilaterally. Dry (non-exudative) AMD is generally managed conservatively. Intravitreal injection of inhibitors of vascular endothelial growth factor (anti-VEGF) is often used in the management of wet (exudative) AMD. Management of cystoid macular oedema (C) is dependent on the cause. Central serous chorioretinopathy (D) usually recovers spontaneously.

13) B

Central serous chorioretinopathy (B) typically occurs in young men, caused by the breakdown of the blood-retinal barrier, resulting in extravasation of fluid from the choroidal vasculature in the subretinal space. Risk factors include stress, steroid use, pregnancy, and sleep apnoea syndrome. On fluorescein angiography, smokestack and ink-blot signs can be seen. Management of central serous chorioretinopathy is typically conservative as the majority resolves spontaneously. Subthreshold photodynamic therapy is sometimes used.

14) D

The brief history in this question describes wet (exudative) AMD. Drusen spots (B) are yellowish deposits between Bruch membrane and the retinal pigment epithelium (RPE). Choroidal neovascularisation (A) defines the exudative stage of AMD. Operculum (D) is not associated with AMD but is seen in macular holes and retinal tears.

15) A

The visual field defect and photopsia described in a patient with marfanoid features are suggestive of a rhegmatogenous retinal detachment (A). The patient does not have risk factors for tractional retinal detachment (B) such as diabetic retinopathy or penetrating posterior segment trauma. Exudative retinal detachment (C) is also unlikely as there are no signs of a choroidal tumour or any inflammatory processes.

16) C

Acquired retinoschisis (C) is a degeneration of the peripheral retina of idiopathic aetiology. It is usually stable but can occasionally lead to retinal detachment. Acquired retinoschisis occurs in up to 5% of the population, and is more commonly seen in individuals with hypermetropia.

17) D

In retinal detachment, fluid accumulates between the retinal pigment epithelium and neurosensory layer (photoreceptor layer). Adhesion of these layers is maintained by a variety of mechanisms including active transport. A number of processes can lead to the collection of subretinal fluid. A break in the retina can lead to the entry of liquefied vitreous into the subretinal space. This is known as rhegmatogenous retinal detachment. Tractional and exudative detachments are other forms of retinal detachment.

18) A

Best disease (A), also known as early-onset vitelliform macular dystrophy, is an autosomal dominant disease. It tends to occur bilaterally and does not significantly affect visual acuity until the cysts rupture, which lead to atrophy of the macula and RPE later on in life. It is the second most common macular dystrophy. The most common macular dystrophy is Stargardt disease (C). It usually starts in adolescence. Juvenile retinoschisis (B) is usually inherited in an X-linked recessive pattern.

19) A

The likely diagnosis is retinoblastoma, the most common primary intraocular malignancy of childhood. It is inherited in around 40% of cases and is associated with mutations of the tumour suppressor gene *RB1*, which is found on chromosome 13 (13q14).

Medical Retina and Vitreoretinal Surgery Answers

20) A
Birdshot chorioretinopathy is a chronic posterior uveitis, which typically manifests as ill-defined cream ovoid lesions in the posterior pole of the fundus. It occurs bilaterally and is also associated with cystoid macular oedema and retinal atrophy. HLA-A29 is a strong genetic risk factor.

21) D
The progressive ophthalmoplegia described in this question, along with signs of deafness and cerebellar ataxia, in a child is suggestive of a mitochondrial disorder called Kearns-Sayre syndrome. It is also associated with cardiac conduction abnormalities, for which an ECG would be necessary to detect. Other signs include "salt and pepper" retinopathy seen on fundoscopy.

22) C
Acute retinal necrosis (ARN) can occur in healthy individuals. At large, HSV (A) is the most likely causative organism in young people, whereas VZV (C) is more commonly seen in older people. ARN can often cause acute onset loss of vision, accompanied by anterior uveitis, scleritis, anterior chamber inflammation, vitritis, peripheral retinal periarteritis and full thickness retinal necrosis. More than 50% of patients develop retinal detachment. Treatment with intravenous aciclovir is important to reduce the risk of second eye involvement.

23) A
Toxoplasmosis in immunocompromised patients or those with sight-threatening, active ocular lesions are treated with systemic prednisolone, pyrimethamine and sulfadiazine (A). Ganciclovir (B) and foscarnet (C) are used in the management of CMV retinitis. Flucytosine (D) is an antifungal agent used in the treatment of endogenous Candida endophthalmitis.

24) B
This patient is likely immunocompromised, suggested by his recent *Pneumocystis* infection. A "pizza pie" appearance and brushfire retinitis are associated with CMV retinitis, which is the most common opportunistic ocular infection in AIDS. CMV spreads to the retina haematogenously, infecting the retinal endothelium and thereafter reaching the retinal cells. Management of CMV retinitis involves medications such as ganciclovir, which can be given through oral, intravenous

or intravitreal routes. Antiretroviral therapy is also a key aspect in the management of CMV retinitis.

25) A
Ethambutol (A), used in the treatment of TB, can cause a central loss of vision and dyschromatopsia. Amiodarone toxicity can lead to progressive binocular vision loss with disc swelling. Alcohol toxicity is associated with photophobia and visual hallucinations. Linezolid toxicity can also cause decreased colour vision, but the patient's past medical history makes ethambutol toxicity more likely.

Chapter 5　Strabismus and Paediatric Ophthalmology Questions

1) What is of the following is the **MOST LIKELY** diagnosis for photophobia and epiphora in a 6-week-old baby?
   A. Congenital cataract
   B. Congenital glaucoma
   C. Retinoblastoma
   D. Retinopathy of prematurity

2) Which of the following is **FALSE**?
   A. Microphthalmos — the entire eye is small and can be associated with other features of ocular dysgenesis
   B. Nanophthalmos — the entire eye is small and structurally abnormal
   C. Buphthalmos — the eye is large as a result of stretching from elevated intraocular pressure
   D. Anophthalmos — there is complete absence of any visible globe structures

3) A 10-year-old boy with a background of joint problems and hearing loss presents with a sudden and painless loss of vision in which he reports seeing a curtain-like shadow coming down across his field of vision. What is the **MOST LIKELY** underlying condition?
   A. Coats disease
   B. Stickler syndrome
   C. Noonan syndrome
   D. Familial exudative vitreoretinopathy

4) What is the average time for neural tube closure?
   A. 28 days
   B. 35 days
   C. 14 days
   D. 7 days

5) What is the embryologic origin of the lenticular anterior epithelium?
   A. Neural crest
   B. Surface ectoderm
   C. Neuroectoderm
   D. Mesoderm

6) Which of the following is **TRUE** about neonatal conjunctivitis?
   A. It can lead to blindness when untreated
   B. Mainly presents in the first week of life
   C. *Neisseria gonorrhoea* is the most common infective cause
   D. Has a 5% incidence in the UK

7) A 2-year-old boy presents with bilateral ecchymosis, weight loss, abdominal distension and left proptosis. Which of the following is the **MOST LIKELY** diagnosis?
   A. Optic nerve glioma
   B. Metastatic neuroblastoma
   C. Wilms tumour
   D. Orbital cellulitis

8) Which of the following is **TRUE** about developmental amblyopia?
   A. Commonly due to media opacity
   B. Is usually bilateral
   C. Occurs in 3–5% of the population
   D. Is usually not treatable

9) Which of the following child is **MOST LIKELY** to develop amblyopia?
   A. 2-year-old with a 1 mm upper lid ptosis in one eye
   B. 12-year-old with left exotropia
   C. 5-year-old with a family history of amblyopia
   D. 4-year-old with uncorrected anisometropia of +2D

10) Which of the following is **FALSE** regarding the current screening criteria for retinopathy of prematurity in the UK?
    A. Babies born at 33 weeks gestational age should be screened
    B. Babies born with a birthweight of 1250 g must be screened
    C. Babies born at 30 weeks gestational age must be screened
    D. Babies born with a birthweight of 1500 g should be screened

11) Which of the following is **NOT** a feature of infantile esotropia?
    A. Small angle of deviation
    B. Onset before 6 months
    C. Alternating fixation
    D. Inferior oblique overaction

12) A 6-year-old boy is referred with gradual deterioration in his right eye. His best corrected visual acuity is 6/12 right eye and 6/5 left eye. He has multiple light brown patches and solitary nodules on his back. A slit lamp examination revealed bilateral tiny pigmented iris nodules and a right optic disc pallor. What is the **MOST LIKELY** diagnosis?
    A. Coats disease
    B. Neurofibromatosis
    C. Tuberous sclerosis
    D. Von Hippel-Lindau syndrome

13) Which of the following is **TRUE** regarding a right 4th nerve palsy?
    A. The left eye is deviated upwards
    B. The squint is better when tilting the head to the right
    C. It is the most common congenital cranial nerve palsy
    D. Microvascular palsies commonly require strabismus surgery

14) Which of the following **DOES NOT** originate from neural crest cells?
    A. Corneal stroma
    B. Dilator pupillae
    C. Iris stroma
    D. Corneal endothelium

15) A 2-month-old baby girl presents with a 1-week history of tearing and mucous discharge from her right eye. On examination, there is a clear bluish mass overlying the lacrimal sac with a reflux of mucoid material from the punctum when gentle pressure is applied over this area. Where is the **MOST LIKELY** level of obstruction?
    A. The valve of Rosenmüller
    B. The lower canaliculus
    C. The valve of Hasner
    D. The lower punctum

16) Which of the following type of exodeviation is **MOST** common?
    A. Pseudoexotropia
    B. Congenital exotropia
    C. Intermittent exotropia
    D. Consecutive exotropia

17) A 2-week-old infant is suspected of having persistent fetal vasculature. Which of the following clinical finding does **NOT** support this diagnosis?
    A. Mittendorf dot
    B. Elongated ciliary processes
    C. Bergmeister papilla
    D. Macrophthalmia

18) Which of the following must be carefully screened for in a child presenting with aniridia?
    A. Phaeochromocytoma
    B. Wilms tumour
    C. Rhabdomyosarcoma
    D. Retinoblastoma

19) Which of the following histological association is **FALSE**?
    A. Multinuclear cells in giant cell arteritis
    B. Rosettes in optic nerve glioma
    C. Peripheral palisades in basal cell carcinoma
    D. Dalen-Fuchs nodules in sympathetic ophthalmia

20) A healthy 12-year-old boy presents with a 2.5 mm anisocoria, which is greater in the light than the dark. What is the most likely underlying cause?
    A. Essential anisocoria
    B. Horner syndrome
    C. Oculomotor nerve palsy
    D. Inadvertent use of topical drops for his younger sibling, who is being treated for amblyopia

21) A cover-uncover test demonstrates no movement of either eye. A subsequent alternate-cover test reveals inward fixation shifts of each eye as the cover is moved. What is the best description of the patient's motility status?
A. Orthophoric, esotropic
B. Orthophoric, exotropic
C. Orthotropic, esophoric
D. Orthotropic, exophoric

22) Which of the following test is **MOST** useful in differentiating a paralytic extraocular disorder from a restrictive disorder?
A. Forced duction test
B. 4 prism dioptre test
C. Double Maddox rod test
D. Parks 3-step test

23) Which muscle is **MOST** effective as a depressor of the eye when it is adducted 51 degrees from the midline?
A. Inferior oblique
B. Inferior rectus
C. Superior oblique
D. Superior rectus

24) Which of the following is **FALSE** regarding the superior rectus muscle?
A. Of the four recti muscles, it has the furthest insertion (7.7 mm) behind the limbus
B. It originates from the upper part of the annulus of Zinn
C. It is innervated by the 3rd cranial (oculomotor) nerve
D. Secondary actions include adduction and extorsion

25) A 76-year-old patient presents with a right 6th nerve palsy and is troubled by diplopia. A large squint is detected on a cover-uncover test. Which of the following prisms would be **MOST** appropriate to address his symptom?
A. Base-out over the right eye
B. Base-in over the right eye
C. Base-out over both eyes
D. Base-in over the left eye and base-out over the right eye

Chapter 5 Strabismus and Paediatric Ophthalmology Answers

1) B
Primary congenital glaucoma usually presents with a classic clinical triad of epiphora, photophobia and blepharospasm that is often noted by parents or a health professional. Buphthalmos (large eyeball size) and corneal haze are other but less common presenting features.

In congenital cataract, there is an absent red reflex and often leukocoria (white pupillary reflex). Other signs include nystagmus, strabismus and an absence of central fixation where the baby is unaware of his/her surroundings or unable to fix and follow.

Retinoblastoma is the most common intraocular malignancy of childhood and accounts for 3% of all childhood cancers. Common signs include leukocoria (most common — 60%) and strabismus (second most common — 20%).

Retinopathy of prematurity results from disordered retinal vascular development in preterm infants and remains a major preventable cause of visual impairment. It is usually detected on screening and treatment of at-risk infants.

2) B
Microphthalmos is a condition in which the eye is small (axial length of <2 standard deviations below the mean for age. This can be further classified into (1) simple or pure microphthalmos (**nanophthalmos**) where the small eye is structurally normal and (2) **complex microphthalmos** where the small eye is associated with other features of dysgenesis (e.g., coloboma and orbital cyst).

3) B
Sudden painless vision loss associated with a curtain-like shadow is characteristic of a retinal detachment. Stickler syndrome is a genetically heterogenous disorder of collagen connective tissue and is the most common inherited cause of retinal detachment in children. Systemic

features include mid-facial hypoplasia, joint hypermobility, early-onset arthritis and deafness.

Coats disease is an idiopathic retinal telangiectasia that most frequently presents in the first decade of life (peak onset at 6–8 years of age) with unilateral visual loss, leukocoria or strabismus. It is associated with intra-/subretinal exudation and frequently exudative retinal detachment.

Noonan syndrome is a genetic disorder characterised by unusual facial features, short stature and head defects and may present with visual loss secondary to ocular complications such as optic nerve hypoplasia or optic disc coloboma.

Familial exudative vitreoretinopathy defines a group of inherited disease with abnormal retina angiogenesis leading to incomplete vascularisation of the peripheral retina. The resultant ischaemia leads to secondary neovascularisation, which then causes traction, exudation and retinal detachment. High myopia may be present but there are usually no associated systemic signs/symptoms.

4) A
Neural tube closure is usually completed by 28 days (4 weeks) from conception. Eye morphogenesis begins with the evagination, or outgrowth, of the optic grooves or sulci. These grooves become outpocketings (known as optic vesicles at this point) as the neural tube closes. The optic vesicles then develop into the optic cup with the inner layer forming the retina and the outer portion forming the retinal pigment epithelium.

5) B
Cells from the surface ectoderm differentiate into cells that form the lens, conjunctival and corneal epithelium, as well as structures associated with tear production and drainage (e.g., meibomian gland, lacrimal gland and nasolacrimal system).

Neuroectoderm gives rise to the retina, optic nerve and epithelial lining of the iris and ciliary body.

The rest of the ocular structures (e.g., extraocular muscles, sclera, trabecular meshwork) originate from the neural crest and mesoderm cells.

6) A
Ophthalmia neonatorum (conjunctivitis of the newborn) is defined as conjunctival inflammation developing within the first month of life. It is

a form of conjunctivitis contracted by newborns during passage through an infected birth canal. The usual infective agents are *Chlamydia trachomatis* and *Neisseria gonorrhoeae* (of which the former is more common). The incidence of neonatal conjunctivitis is <1% in the UK. Blindness can rapidly ensue if this is left untreated.

7) B

Neuroblastoma is one of the most common childhood malignancies. It is a poorly differentiated neoplasm derived from neural crest cells that typically affects infants and children <5 years of age. More than 50% of patients have metastatic disease at presentation, which carries a very poor prognosis. Orbital metastases may be bilateral and typically present with painless proptosis accompanied by a superior orbital mass and lid ecchymosis.

Optic nerve glioma is a slow-growing astrocytoma that typically affects children (mean age of 6 years). Prognosis is variable and approximately 30% have associated neurofibromatosis (NF) type I. Patients may present with slowly progressive unilateral visual loss and proptosis. Systemic signs and symptoms are usually absent unless associated with NF type I.

Wilms tumour (nephroblastoma) is a malignant tumour that develops in the kidney. It may be part of the WARG syndrome, which is a rare genetic syndrome in which affected children are predisposed to develop **W**ilms tumour, **A**niridia, **G**enitourinary anomalies and mental **R**etardation. Aniridia is typically the first noticeable sign of the WAGR syndrome.

Orbital cellulitis refers to inflammation of ocular tissue behind the orbital septum. It is most commonly secondary to an acute spread of infection into the orbit from either the adjacent sinuses or haematologically. It usually presents with proptosis, painful eye movement, and redness and swelling of the eyelid. Patients may have systemic symptoms such as fever and lethargy. Without proper treatment, it can lead to serious consequences including permanent vision loss and even death.

8) C

Amblyopia is a relatively common disorder and a major cause of visual impairment in children. It represents an insult to the visual system during the critical period of development whereby an ocular pathology (e.g., high refractive error, anisometropia, strabismus) interferes with normal cortical visual development. Approximately 3–5% of children are affected by amblyopia. Bilateral amblyopia is less common than unilateral amblyopia. The most common causes of unilateral amblyopia are strabismus and anisometropia, or a combination of the two. The aetiologies of amblyopia can be remembered with the following mnemonic: **S.O.S** — **S**pectacles (anisometropia or high refractive error), **O**cclusion (media opacity or any ocular pathology) and **S**trabismus. Active treatment (e.g., patching, pharmacologic agents) can often improve the residual visual deficit, especially if instigated at an early stage.

9) D
As discussed in Question 8, the most common causes of unilateral amblyopia are strabismus and anisometropia, or a combination of two. In anisometropic amblyopia, this may result from a difference as little as 1 dioptre. The more ametropic eye experiences a mild form of visual deprivation due to a blurred image.

The risk of developing amblyopia diminishes as the child approaches 8–10 years of age. As a corollary to this, the depth of amblyopia is typically less severe the older the child is at the time of onset of the amblyogenic factor.

An upper lid ptosis of 1 mm is minimal, and unless severe and covering the pupil entirely, is insufficient to cause stimulus deprivation amblyopia.

A positive family history of strabismus increases the risk of amblyopia in the child but does not confer the same risk as amblyogenic factors such as strabismus and anisometropia.

10) A
The current inclusion criteria for screening for retinopathy of prematurity (ROP) in the UK is:

- Babies born <32 weeks or ≤1501 g birthweight **should** be screened for ROP. One criterion has to be met for inclusion.
- Babies born <31 weeks or ≤1251 g birthweight **must** be screened for ROP. One criterion has to be met for inclusion.

11) A
Infantile esotropia (also known as congenital or early onset esotropia) is an idiopathic esotropia developing within the first 6 months of life in an otherwise normal infant with no significant refractive error or limitation

of ocular movements. The angle is usually fairly large (>30 prism dioptres) and stable. Fixation is mostly alternating in the primary position. There is also often an associated inferior oblique overaction, which may develop subsequently, most commonly at 2 years of age.

12) B

Neurofibromatosis type I (NF1), also known as von Recklinghausen disease, is the most common phacomatosis (alongside tuberous sclerosis, Von Hippel-Lindau syndrome, Sturge-Weber syndrome). Inheritance is autosomal dominant and NF1 is caused by mutations in a gene called *NF1*, which is found on chromosome 17. The presence of optic nerve glioma and Lisch nodules (iris hamartomas which present as tiny pigmented iris nodules) are important ophthalmic diagnostic signs. The former typically occurs in young children and may present with painless proptosis and optic atrophy (and hence optic disc pallor). Systemic features include neurofibromas (solitary nodules), café-au-lait (light-brown patches), axillary/inguinal freckles and skeletal abnormalities.

13) C

The 4th (trochlear) cranial nerve (CN IV) supplies only the superior oblique muscle, which elevates, intorts and abducts the globe. CN IV palsy is the most common **congenital** cranial nerve palsy (approximately 75% of all cases are congenital). A right CN IV is characterised by ipsilateral hypertropia ("right over left") in the primary position. The hypertropia will improve with abduction of the hypertropic eye and head tilt to the contralateral side. Microvascular palsies commonly resolve spontaneously without requiring strabismus surgery.

14) B

Neural crest cells migrate between the lens and corneal epithelium (both of which originate from the surface ectoderm) to form the corneal endothelium and stroma.

Both dilator and sphincter pupillae muscles of the iris are derived from the **neuroectoderm**. The stroma of the iris and ciliary body, on the other hand, develops from **neural crest cells** that migrate into this area.

15) C

Nasolacrimal duct obstruction (NLDO) is a blockage of the lacrimal drainage system and is congenital in the majority of children. It occurs approximately in 5% of newborn infants and the rate of spontaneous resolution is estimated to be 90% within the first year of life. Affected infants typically present with a history of epiphora and mucous discharge. A mucocoele often forms within the lacrimal sac as a result of congenital NLDO and this is seen as a bluish, cystic mass just below the medial canthus in the area of the nasolacrimal sac. In congenital NLDO, the blockage occurs most commonly at the valve of Hasner at the distal end of the duct due to non-canalisation of this portion of the nasolacrimal duct.

16) C

Intermittent exotropia is the most common exodeviation. Presentation is often at around 2 years and usually begins as an exophoria, which breaks down to exotropia under conditions of visual inattention, fatigue or ill health.

Pseudoexotropia is not a true strabismus disorder and is the result of certain morphological features of the face, which result in the false appearance of eyes to be drifted outwards. A common example of this is hypertelorism, in which the eyes are widely set apart.

Congenital exotropia is an uncommon entity. Consecutive exotropia develops spontaneously in an amblyopic eye, or more frequently following surgical correction of an esodeviation.

17) D

Persistent fetal vasculature (PFV) (also known as persistent hyperplastic primary vitreous) is a spectrum of disease that can present with a wide range of signs and symptoms, ranging from no clinical effect to severe morbidity. This condition arises from the failure of the hyaloid vasculature to undergo normal programmed involution.

PFV is divided into three subcategories: anterior, posterior, or a combination of the two. In anterior PFV, remnants of the tunica vasculosa lentis fail to regress and a Mittendorf dot can be seen. This is a small, circular opacity on the posterior lens capsule, classically nasal in location where the hyaloid artery attaches anteriorly. Elongated ciliary body processes are also commonly seen in anterior PFV.

In posterior PFV, there may be a persistence of a small part of the posterior portion of the hyaloid artery, which is referred to as a Bergmeister papilla. This anomaly generally takes the form of a veil-like structure or a fingerlike projection extending anteriorly from the surface of the optic nerve head.

Microphthalmia (rather than macrophthalmia) is associated with both anterior and posterior types of PFV and is often one of the first signs of PFV in an infant.

18) B

Aniridia is a rare genetic disorder in which there is a variable degree of hypoplasia or absence of iris associated with other ocular features. It may present from birth or arise progressively over time. It is important to instigate thorough systemic screening as it may have life-threatening associations (e.g., Wilms tumour).

In the vast majority (two thirds) of cases, aniridia occurs in isolation without systemic involvement due to dominantly inherited mutations or deletions of the paired box gene-6 (*PAX6*). In a minority of cases, it can occur sporadically as part of the WAGR (**W**ilms tumour, **A**niridia, **G**enitourinary anomalies, mental **R**etardation) contiguous gene syndrome in which the adjacent *PAX6* and Wilms tumour (*WT1*) genes are both deleted. Children with sporadic aniridia have about a 33% chance of developing Wilms' tumour.

Phaeochromocytoma is found in Von Hippel-Lindau disease.

Rhabdomyosarcoma is the most common primary orbital malignancy in children but is still a rare condition and does not have any specific systemic association.

Retinoblastoma is the most common primary intraocular malignancy of childhood and accounts for about 3% of all childhood cancers. Heritable retinoblastoma accounts for 40% and has a predisposition to non-ocular cancers such as pinealoblastoma ("trilateral retinoblastoma"), osteosarcoma and melanoma.

19) B

A feature of retinoblastoma includes the formation of Flexner-Wintersteiner and Homer-Wright rosettes, which are formations of retinal differentiation. These rosettes are also seen in other neuroblastic tumours but not optic nerve glioma.

20) D

Essential (physiologic) anisocoria is the most common cause of unequal pupil sizes, affecting up to 20% of the population. It is a benign condition with a difference in pupil size of ≤1 mm. The degree of anisocoria is equal in light and dark.

Horner syndrome (oculosympathetic palsy) is classically described by the triad of ptosis, miosis and anhidrosis. The anisocoria in Horner syndrome is greater in the dark than in the light due to a defect in the pupillary dilator response resulting from lesions along the sympathetic trunk.

Oculomotor nerve (CN III) palsy varies in presentation and aetiology but rarely presents as isolated mydriasis. Associated signs include ptosis, an ipsilateral "down and out" gaze, and a loss of accommodation. Anisocoria due to CN III palsy is greater in the light than in the dark due to a parasympathetic defect, resulting in an abnormal pupil that is larger and unable to constrict in response to a light stimulus.

Accidental use of pharmacological mydriatics (e.g., cyclopentolate, atropine) can also result in anisocoria that is greater in the light than in the dark. These topical agents (which also have cycloplegic properties) are often used to pharmacologically penalise the non-amblyopic (better) eye in the treatment of amblyopia. In contrast to CN III palsy, patients are often otherwise asymptomatic.

21) D
There is no manifest deviation (tropia) on the cover-uncover test but there is a latent exodeviation (phoria) on the alternate-cover test.

22) A
The forced duction test is a test of extraocular muscle (EOM) function that is useful in differentiating between EOM paresis and restriction. The anaesthetised conjunctiva is grasped with forceps and an attempt is made to move the eye in the direction where the movement is restricted. In a restrictive disorder, it will not be possible to induce a passive movement of the eyeball whereas the converse is true for a paretic disorder.

23) C
When the globe is adducted 51 degrees, the visual axis coincides with the line of pull of the superior oblique muscle. In this position it can act only as a depressor, and hence, this is the best position to test the action of the superior oblique muscle. The main sequela of superior oblique weakness is seen as the failure of depression in adduction.

24) D
Secondary actions of the superior rectus muscle are adduction and **intorsion**.

25) C

The apex (which is the opposite direction to the base) of a prism should always point towards the direction of the deviated eye. In a right 6th nerve palsy, there is right esotropia due to weakness of the lateral rectus muscle and secondary overaction of the ipsilateral medial rectus muscle. An esotropia would therefore require a base-out (i.e., apex facing inwards) for correction.

For small angle squints, the correction can be placed over the affected eye only. However, for large angle squints, it is better treated by splitting the power of the prisms between the two eyes. In the case of an esodeviation, a base-out prism is placed over each eye (and vice versa for exodeviation). For example, a 21 prism dioptre (PD) right esotropia can be treated with 11 and 10 PD base-out prisms placed over the right and left eye, respectively.

Chapter 6 Neuro-ophthalmology Questions

1) Which of the following represents results expected from visual evoked potential (VEP) in optic neuropathy?
   A. Prolongation of latency and decreased amplitude
   B. Prolongation of latency and increased amplitude
   C. Reduction of latency and decreased amplitude
   D. Reduction of latency and increased amplitude

2) Which of the following is a cause of consecutive optic atrophy?
   A. Optic neuritis
   B. Trauma
   C. Retinitis pigmentosa
   D. Chronic papilloedema

3) Which of the following signs may **NOT** be seen in primary optic atrophy?
   A. Flat white disc with clear margins
   B. Thinning of the retinal nerve fibre layer
   C. Reduction in the number of small bloods vessels on the disc surface
   D. Obscuration of the lamina cribrosa

4) Temporal pallor of the optic nerve head is most commonly seen in which of the following?
   A. Demyelinating optic neuritis
   B. Lesion of the optic chiasm
   C. Chronic papilloedema
   D. Retinitis pigmentosa

5) Which of the following signs may be seen in the "established" stage of papilloedema?
   A. Drusen deposits on disc surface
   B. Severely impaired visual acuity
   C. Enlarged blind spot
   D. Grey optic disc

6) A 50-year-old-woman presents with a sudden worsening of right vision after a warm shower, which has now resulted in painful eye movements in the affected eye. Which of the following signs are you likely to see on ophthalmoscopy?
   A. Neuroretinitis
   B. Retrobulbar neuritis
   C. Papillitis
   D. Optic atrophy

7) A 54-year-old gentleman presents with a sudden onset painless loss of vision in his right eye upon waking this morning. He has longstanding type 2 diabetes mellitus, hypertension and hypercholesterolaemia. Which of the following statements regarding this diagnosis is **TRUE**?
   A. Dyschromatopsia is usually proportional to the level of visual impairment
   B. Disc swelling persists for months after onset
   C. Disc pallor is rare after onset
   D. Most common visual defect is superior altitudinal

8) A 72-year-old-gentleman presents with a right-sided headache that is worse on palpation. This is associated with a cramp-like pain on chewing, fever, weight loss and proximal joint stiffness. He now complains of double vision. Which of the following is **NOT** an ocular manifestation of the suspected diagnosis in this patient?
   A. Ocular ischaemic syndrome
   B. Cilioretinal artery occlusion
   C. Central retinal artery occlusion
   D. Non-arteritic anterior ischaemic optic neuropathy

9) Which of the following facts regarding posterior ischaemic optic neuropathy (PION) is **TRUE**?
   A. There are broadly speaking three different types — arteritic, non-arteritic and infectious
   B. PION may develop perioperatively, especially in surgery involving the heart and spine
   C. PION is more common than anterior ischaemic optic neuropathy
   D. PION is caused by ischaemia of the posterior ciliary artery

10) Which of the following statements regarding Leber hereditary optic neuropathy (LHON) is **FALSE**?
    A. It is a rare ganglion cell degeneration, affecting the papillomacular bundle in particular
    B. It is caused by maternally inherited mitochondrial DNA point mutations, usually in the MT-ND4 gene
    C. There is often no relative afferent pupillary defect (RAPD)
    D. Peripheral vision is usually preserved

11) A 42-year-old lady presents with a 2-week history of worsening morning headaches, persistent nausea with occasional vomiting and transient "greying-out" of vision. Which of the following investigations is **least** likely to be indicated?
    A. B-scan ultrasonography
    B. Lumbar puncture
    C. CT venogram
    D. Chest X-ray

12) A 50-year-old-gentleman presents with a 1-week history of a persistent right-sided headache. On examination you note he has slight ptosis of the right eye and mild anisocoria with the right pupil measuring 2 mm and the left measuring 6 mm. Which of the following investigations is **most** likely to be indicated?
    A. CT spine
    B. CT angiography
    C. CT neck
    D. CT chest

13) Which of the following results indicates a positive Horner pupil when using apraclonidine 0.5%?
    A. The affected pupil will dilate, the normal pupil is unaffected. Ptosis improves.
    B. The affected pupil will dilate, the normal pupil will dilate. Ptosis is unaffected.
    C. The affected pupil remains the same, the normal pupil will dilate. Ptosis is unaffected.
    D. The affected pupil remains the same, the normal pupil is unaffected. Ptosis improves.

14) A 21-year-old female presents with a blurring of near vision and notices asymmetrical pupils. On examination the left pupil is larger than the right and has a sluggish response to direct and consensual light reflex. On a slit lamp examination you note vermiform movements of the pupillary border on the left. Which of the following investigations is most helpful in confirming the diagnosis?
    A. Apraclonidine 0.5%
    B. Pilocarpine 0.1%
    C. Cocaine 4%
    D. Observation

15) A 54-year-old has bilateral, small irregular pupils, which respond poorly to light but retain a normal near reflex. Which of the following tests is **NOT** indicated to investigate the suspected underlying cause?
    A. HbA1c
    B. Syphilis serology
    C. FBC and LFTs
    D. HIV serology

16) Which of the following is **NOT** typically a cause of light-near dissociation?
    A. Adie pupil
    B. Argyll Robertson pupil
    C. Parinaud syndrome
    D. Brown syndrome

17) Which of the following is typically **NOT** an ophthalmic feature in pituitary adenomas?
    A. Colour desaturation across the vertical midline
    B. Optic atrophy
    C. Papilloedema
    D. Bitemporal superior quadrantanopia is the first defect

18) A 58-year-old complains of double vision and a headache. On examination you note profound ptosis of the left eye with abduction and depression in the primary position. There is limited adduction and elevation of the left eye. The right eye is normal. The left pupil is dilated and has poor response to accommodation. Which of the following investigations is indicated in the first instance?
    A. HbA1c
    B. CT angiography
    C. ESR
    D. MRI brain and orbits

19) Which of the following regions does the initiation for horizontal saccades originate?
    A. Premotor cortex
    B. Paramedian pontine reticular formation
    C. Medial longitudinal fasciculus
    D. Parieto-occipto-temporal junction

20) A 49-year-old woman presents with double vision. On examination you note that on right gaze she is able to abduct the right eye, but the left eye is unable to adduct. This is accompanied by ataxic nystagmus of the right eye when it is abducted. On left gaze there is limitation of right adduction and nystagmus of the abducted left eye. Where is the lesion?
    A. Cerebral cortex with raised ICP
    B. Bilateral paramedian pontine reticular formation lesion
    C. Bilateral medial longitudinal fasciculus lesion
    D. Bilateral medial rectus lesion

21) A 32-year-old lady with generalised fatigue and peripheral muscle weakness complains of double vision. On examination there is asymmetrical bilateral ptosis and complex ophthalmoplegia causing vertical diplopia. Which of the following tests is least likely to aid diagnosis?
   A. Tensilon test
   B. Schirmer test
   C. Ice pack test
   D. Antibody test

22) A 58-year-old gentleman presents with difficulty walking, dysarthria and bilateral facial wasting with hollow cheeks. You also note some frontal baldness on examination. Which of the following ophthalmic features does **NOT** typically appear in this condition?
   A. Cataract
   B. Ptosis
   C. Hypermetropia
   D. Glaucoma

23) A 14-year-old presents with gradual onset bilateral ptosis. On examination, he has complex ophthalmoplegia affecting both eyes. His ECG reveals a prolonged QTc interval. Which of the following findings would you expect on fundoscopy?
   A. "Salt and pepper" retinopathy
   B. Retinitis pigmentosa
   C. Bull's-eye maculopathy
   D. Roth spots

24) A 39-year-old woman presents with diplopia associated with nausea and headache after recently returning from a trip in Thailand. She suffered from traveller's diarrhoea recently but is otherwise fit and well. On examination, she is ataxic and has hyporeflexia. Which of the following is most likely to show an abnormality?
   A. Anti-GQ1b
   B. Fundoscopy
   C. MRI Head
   D. p-ANCA

25) Which of the following is **NOT** an ophthalmic manifestation of neurofibromatosis type I?
   A. Glaucoma
   B. Prominent corneal nerves
   C. Cataract
   D. Retinal astrocytoma

Chapter 6 Neuro-ophthalmology Answers

1) A

A visual evoked potential (VEP) test records electrical activity of the visual cortex when the retina is stimulated. This is often via flashing a light (flash VEP) or displaying a black-and-white checkerboard pattern that periodically reverses polarity (pattern VEP). Optic neuropathy would cause both an increased latent period and reduced amplitude in response to the stimuli.

2) C

Optic atrophy is the result of axonal degeneration in the pathway of the optic nerve between the retina and the lateral geniculate body. Causes of optic atrophy can be subdivided into primary, secondary and consecutive.

Cause	Site of Lesion	Examples
Primary	From retrolaminar portion of the optic nerve to lateral geniculate body	— Optic neuritis — Hereditary optic neuropathies — Compressive masses (e.g., tumour) — Trauma
Secondary	Optic nerve head	— Chronic papilloedema — Papillitis — Anterior ischaemic optic neuropathy
Consecutive	Inner retina	— Retinitis pigmentosa

There is also glaucomatous optic atrophy.

3) D

The following table helps to identify which signs may be seen in the different classifications of optic atrophy, in particular, primary versus secondary optic atrophy.

Optic Atrophy Classification	Signs
Primary	— Flat white disc with clear margins — Reduction in number of small blood vessels on disc surface — Thinning of retinal nerve fibre layer
Secondary	— Raised white-grey disc with poorly defined margins (due to gliosis) — Obscuration of the lamina cribrosa — Reduction in the number of blood vessels on the disc surface — Peripapillary circumferential retinochoroidal folds
Consecutive	— Usually signs are related to cause (e.g., retinitis pigmentosa) — Disc usually appears waxy

4) A

Demyelinating optic neuritis causes primary optic neuropathy and typically causes temporal pallor of the optic nerve head (indicating atrophy of the papillomacular bundle). Lesions of the optic chiasm give band atrophy, whereby there is nasal and temporal pallor as it involves fibres entering the optic disc nasally and temporally. Chronic papilloedema causes signs of secondary optic atrophy (see previous table).

5) C

The stages of papilloedema are outlined as follows:

Stage	Features
Early	— Mild disc hyperaemia — Preservation of the optic cup

(Continued)

(*Continued*)

Stage	Features
Established	— Severe disc hyperaemia — Absence of physiological cup — Venous engorgement, cotton wool spots, peripapillary flame haemorrhages — Enlarged blind spot
Chronic	— No cotton wool spots/haemorrhages — Visual fields begin to constrict — Drusen-like deposits may be present on the disc surface
Atrophic	— Visual acuity is severely impaired — Optic discs appear grey-white, elevated and with indistinct margins

Absence of spontaneous venous pulsation is typically an early sign of papilloedema but is an unreliable sign as it may be identifiable in normal individuals.

6) B

This is a case of multiple sclerosis (MS), which is an idiopathic demyelinating disease involving the central nervous system white matter. The presentation describes symptoms of optic neuritis (common feature of MS), which includes reduction of visual acuity in one eye (including loss of colour vision) and pain behind the eye, which is exacerbated by eye movements. The Uhthoff phenomenon is a transient feature in MS, which refers to a sudden worsening of vision when there is an increase in body temperature. Optic neuritis can be classified into aetiology (i.e., demyelinating, infectious, non-infectious) or according to ophthalmoscope findings as outlined below:

Retrobulbar Neuritis	Optic disc appears normal — Most common finding in demyelinating optic neuritis
Papillitis	Hyperaemia and oedema of optic disc — Usually in children

(Continued)

Neuroretinitis	Papillitis + inflammation of the retinal nerve fibre layer and a macular star figure — Least common type, rarely manifestation of demyelination — Cat-scratch fever is responsible for most cases

7) A

This is a case of non-arteritic anterior ischaemic optic neuropathy (NAION), which is caused by occlusion of the short posterior ciliary arteries. Risk factors are similar to those for cardiovascular diseases (e.g., hypertension, hypercholesteremia, diabetes mellitus). It may also occur following cataract surgery. Signs include the following:

- Visual acuity is usually impaired at least moderately (may be preserved in approximately one third)
- Most common visual field defect is inferior altitudinal
- Dyschromatopsia is usually proportional to the level of visual impairment
- Fundoscopy findings in the acute presentation may include hyperaemic disc swelling and peripapillary splinter haemorrhages
- Disc swelling gradually resolves and pallor ensues 3–6 weeks after onset

8) D

This case describes giant cell arteritis (GCA), a large vessel vasculitis that is most commonly seen in the elderly population and is characterised by scalp tenderness, jaw claudication, non-specific systemic signs (e.g., fever, weight loss, malaise) and is associated with polymyalgia rheumatica in approximately 50% of the patients. Ocular manifestations include cilioretinal artery occlusion, central retinal artery occlusion and ocular ischaemic syndrome (rare). The most common manifestation is arteritic anterior ischaemic optic neuropathy, which typically presents with sudden, profound unilateral visual loss (can be preceded by double vision). Treatment aims at preventing further visual loss in the unaffected eye with high-dose steroids (50–60 mg) for 4 weeks, after which a slow weaning dose is commenced.

9) B

PION is much less common than its anterior counterpart. It is caused by ischaemia of the surrounding pial capillary plexus (supplied by the ophthalmic artery). The diagnosis is usually that of exclusion after ruling out other causes of retrobulbar neuropathy. There are broadly speaking 3 different types (see table below): operative, arteritic and non-arteritic.

Operative	Usually occurs with surgeries involving the heart and spine — Risk factors are anaemia and intraoperative hypovolaemia
Arteritic	Associated with GCA
Non-arteritic	Associated with cardiovascular risk factors

10) C

LHON is a rare ganglion cell degeneration preferentially affecting the papillomacular bundle. It is caused by maternally inherited mitochondrial DNA point mutations. Although it typically affects males (aged 15–35 years), females can also be affected. Typical symptoms include painless acute loss of central vision in one eye (the contralateral eye becomes affected within weeks/months). There is often a RAPD and visual field defects tend to be central scotomas, with preservation of peripheral vision. There is no known treatment; management options revolve around conservative measures such as avoiding dietary deficiencies and smoking cessation.

11) D

The symptoms described are in keeping with raised intracranial pressure (ICP). In such cases, visual symptoms rarely occur in the early stages. Visual manifestations include a transient loss of vision and double vision (usually due to an abducens nerve palsy, a false localising sign). Fundoscopy may reveal papilloedema (bilateral disc swelling secondary to raised ICP). Below are some investigations indicated for papilloedema and their significance.

B-scan Ultrasonography	Helps distinguish between true papilloedema and other causes of a swollen optic disc — This technique measures the diameter of the optic nerve sheath, which is distended in papilloedema
CT Head/MRI Head	To exclude space-occupying lesion
CT Venogram/ MRI Venogram	To exclude cerebral venous sinus thrombosis
Lumbar Puncture	To rule out intracranial infection — **NB** this cannot be done if there is a space-occupying lesion

12) B

This is a case of Horner syndrome. This syndrome is defined by ptosis, miosis and anhidrosis of the affected side. Causes are summarised in the table below:

Classification of Horner Syndrome	Location of Pathology
Central (1st Order Neurone)	• Hypothalamus • Brainstem • Spinal Cord
Preganglionic (2nd Order Neurone)	• Cervical spine injury • Brachial plexus • Thyroid lesions • Apical lung lesions
Postganglionic (3rd Order Neurone)	• Superior cervical ganglion • Internal carotid artery • Skull base lesions • Cavernous sinus lesions • Cluster headaches (can cause permanent or transient Horner)

The mainstay of investigation is imaging; a CT or MR angiography examining the region from the aortic arch to the circle of Willis will facilitate the exclusion of neck (including carotid), apical lung, thyroid and skull base lesions. MR may be utilised if greater soft tissue definition is required, such as to exclude a brainstem stroke. Plain X-rays and carotid ultrasound imaging have limited utility. In particular, painful Horner syndrome should raise the possibility of a carotid dissection.

13) A

Apraclonidine is commonly used to confirm a diagnosis of Horner syndrome (it is highly sensitive and specific). The following will be noted in a Horner pupil:

- A Horner pupil will dilate but a normal pupil is essentially unaffected
- The ptosis commonly also improves

This is primarily due to the upregulation of alpha-1 receptors in the denervated dilator pupillae.

Remember that apraclonidine is used to confirm the diagnosis whereas phenylephrine 1% or hydroxyamphetamine 1% are used to differentiate a preganglionic lesion from a postganglionic lesion.

14) B

This patient has a left Adie pupil. An Adie pupil is a tonic, dilated pupil with sluggish or absent direct reflex test. Instilling pilocarpine 0.1% to both eyes is usually used to confirm an Adie pupil and it will result in a constriction of the abnormal pupil (via denervation hypersensitivity phenomenon). Typically, no treatment is necessary; reading glasses may be advised for near vision, and sunglasses to improve photophobia.

15) D

This case describes Argyll Robertson pupils where both pupils are small and irregular and do not typically respond to light but are able to constrict upon accommodation (light-near dissociation). Typical causes include neurosyphilis, diabetes mellitus (HbA1c) and alcoholism (FBC for MCV and LFTs).

16) D

Light-near dissociation describes the phenomenon whereby the pupillary light reflex is affected but near reflex (accommodation) is spared. Brown syndrome is a condition involving mechanical restriction, typically of the superior oblique tendon. It does not cause light-near dissociation. The table below summarises the main causes of light-near dissociation and their differentiating features.

Condition	Aetiology	Relative Size to Unaffected Pupil	Reactive to Light	Reactive to Accommodation
Marcus Gunn Pupil	RAPD due to an optic nerve lesion	Same	Less than unaffected pupil	Yes
Adie Pupil	Damage to the parasympathetic ciliary ganglion	Dilated	Slow and incomplete	Yes
Argyll Robertson Pupil	Damage to the pretectal area neurons from neurosyphilis	Constricted	No	Yes
Parinaud Syndrome	Compression of the medial longitudinal fasciculus by a pineal gland tumour	Both pupils are mid-dilated	No	Yes

17) C

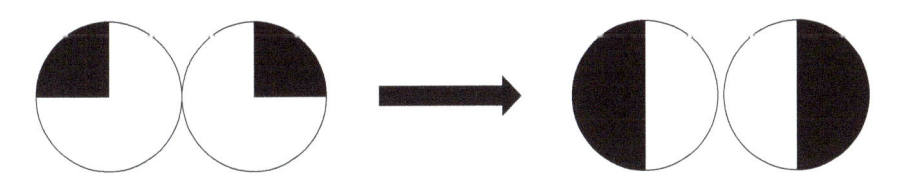

Pituitary adenomas may present with headaches, but diagnostic delay is common as there are typically no features of raised ICP. Colour desaturation across the vertical midline of the uniocular visual field is an early sign of chiasmal compression. Optic atrophy is present in roughly half of the patients. Papilloedema is rare. Bitemporal superior quadrantanopia initially occurs (lower nasal optic nerve fibres are affected first by chiasmal tumours, these are responsible for the upper temporal quadrants of vision) before progressing to a bitemporal hemianopia (see figure).

18) B

This patient has a "surgical", painful 3rd cranial nerve (CN III) palsy. This nerve innervates all of the extraocular muscles except superior oblique (CN IV) and lateral rectus (CN VI). This presents with profound ptosis due to weakness of the levator muscle. In the primary position, the eye is abducted and depressed ("down and out") due to unopposed action of the lateral rectus and superior oblique muscle.

Involvement of the pupil may help to differentiate a medical CN III palsy from a surgical one. Surgical lesions such as a posterior communicating artery aneurysm typically involve the pupil as they compress the pial blood vessels and the superficial pupillary fibres. Medical lesions such as diabetes tend to spare the pupil as they involve the central vasa nervorum. However, it is important to note that these principles are not infallible as pupillary involvement may be seen in "medical" lesions, while pupillary sparing does not rule out an aneurysm or other compressive lesion.

In this case, a CT angiography is the most appropriate first-line investigation to exclude an expanding aneurysm. An MRI brain scan and orbits can subsequently be useful for exclusion of brainstem tumours/strokes, cavernous sinus or orbital apex lesion.

19) A

Saccades allow for fixation from one target to another. There are separate horizontal and vertical pathways — the horizontal pathway is better mapped than the vertical one. Initiation occurs in the premotor cortex (frontal eye fields), which then passes to the contralateral paramedian pontine reticular formation (PPRF). From there impulses pass to the ipsilateral CN VI nucleus and indirectly (via medial longitudinal fasciculus [MLF]) to the contralateral CN III to mediate medial rectus movement.

20) C

This describes a case of bilateral MLF lesion. The MLF is responsible for conjugate horizontal gaze as it allows ipsilateral abduction (mediated by ipsilateral lateral rectus via CN VI) and contralateral adduction (mediated by contralateral medial rectus via CN III). A lesion in the MLF results in internuclear ophthalmoplegia (INO). In a unilateral INO, there is defective adduction of the eye on the SAME side of the lesion with nystagmus of the CONTRALATERAL eye (which would be abducted). In a bilateral INO, the same defect is demonstrated in both right and left gaze. Gaze to the side of the lesion would be NORMAL. Lesions in the PPRF result in ipsilateral horizontal gaze palsy with an inability to look in the direction of the lesion.

21) B

This describes a patient with myasthenia gravis, which typically manifests in the third decade and causes proximal muscle weakness and ocular manifestations including ptosis and diplopia. It is an autoimmune disease caused by anti-acetylcholine receptor (anti-AChR) antibodies in most cases. The symptoms tend to worsen at the end of the day (fatigability). Ptosis is insidious, bilateral and usually asymmetrical. Diplopia tends to be vertical and patients can present with complex ophthalmoplegias (i.e., not limited to one extraocular muscle). Investigations for myasthenia include:

- **Ice pack test**: cold inhibits breakdown of acetylcholine by acetylcholinesterase, therefore resulting in an improvement of ptosis
- **Antibody testing**: anti-AChR antibodies are present in the majority of cases. Anti-MuSK (muscle-specific kinase) antibodies may be present in those negative for anti-AChR
- **Tensilon test**: Edrophonium (a short acting anticholinesterase) given intravenously will result in transient improvement in symptoms
- **Electromyography**
- **Muscle biopsy**: this will reveal neuromuscular junction antibodies
- **Thoracic imaging**: may be necessary to exclude a thymoma
- **Thyroid function testing**: to screen for associated autoimmune thyroid disease

22) D

This patient has signs typical of myotonic dystrophy. Ophthalmic features include:

Common	Uncommon
• Early-onset cataract • Ptosis • Hypermetropia	• Motility dysfunction (e.g., strabismus) • Light-near dissociation • Optic atrophy • Pigmentary retinopathy

23) A

Kearns-Sayre syndrome is a mitochondrial myopathy associated with mitochondrial DNA deletions. Presentation occurs by the second decade. The classic triad is of chronic progressive external ophthalmoplegia (ptosis and slowly progressive bilateral ocular immobility), cardiac conduction abnormalities and pigmentary retinopathy ("salt and pepper" appearance).

24) A

This describes a case of Miller Fisher syndrome, which is an acute polyneuropathy that typically affects extraocular muscles. It typically presents with a triad of ophthalmoplegia, areflexia and ataxia. In the majority of patients anti-GQ1b antibodies are present.

25) C

Neurofibromatosis (NF) is a common phakomatosis affecting cell growth in neural tissues. NF1 is more common than NF2. Ophthalmic manifestations of NF1 include:

o Eyelid plexiform neurofibroma: results in a S-shaped deformity of the upper lid
o Orbital tumours: such as optic nerve glioma
o Iris lesions: Lisch nodules
o Prominent corneal nerves
o Glaucoma
o Fundus lesions: choroidal naevi and hamartomata, retinal astrocytoma

Cataract is a feature predominantly seen in NF2.

Chapter 7 Ocular Adnexal and Orbital Disease Questions

1) Which one of the following bone is **NOT** part of the orbital floor?
   A. Zygoma
   B. Maxilla
   C. Lesser wing of the sphenoid
   D. Palatine

2) Which one of the following bone is **NOT** part of the medial wall of the orbit?
   A. Maxilla
   B. Lacrimal
   C. Ethmoid
   D. Frontal

3) Which of the following regarding the superior orbital fissure is **FALSE**?
   A. It is found between the greater and lesser wings of the sphenoid bone
   B. The lacrimal nerve passes through it and lies outside the annulus of Zinn
   C. The ophthalmic vein passes through it and lies inside the annulus of Zinn
   D. The abducens nerve passes through it and lies inside the annulus of Zinn

4) Which one of the following would **NOT** give rise to axial proptosis?
   A. Cavernous haemangioma
   B. Lacrimal gland tumour
   C. Optic nerve glioma
   D. Optic nerve meningioma

5) Which of the following is **NOT** typically used to differentiate between a restrictive and neurological ophthalmoplegia?
   A. Forced duction test
   B. Differential intraocular pressure test
   C. Saccadic eye movements
   D. Slit lamp ophthalmoscopy

6) Which one of the following is **NOT** typically seen in thyroid eye disease?
   A. Optic neuropathy
   B. Kocher sign
   C. Restrictive myopathy
   D. Phthisis bulbi

7) Which one of the following is/are common causative agent(s) in bacterial orbital cellulitis?
   A. *Streptococcus pyogenes*
   B. *Staphylococcus aureus*
   C. *Streptococcus pneumoniae*
   D. All of the above

8) Which of the following is **FALSE** regarding a direct carotid-cavernous fistula?
   A. A high flow shunt results in blood passing directly from the carotid artery into the cavernous sinus
   B. Patients may present with a triad of pulsatile proptosis, conjunctival chemosis, and a whooshing noise in the head
   C. Spontaneous rupture of an intracavernous sinus aneurysm is the most common cause for the formation of carotid-cavernous fistulae
   D. Most direct carotid-cavernous sinus fistulae are not life threatening

9) Which of the following is **NOT** a feature of a dacryops?
   A. A protruding, round cystic lesion
   B. It protrudes into the inferior fornix
   C. Cyst of the lacrimal gland
   D. Develops from an obstructed duct

Ocular Adnexal and Orbital Disease Questions

10) Which of the following does **NOT** traverse the annulus of Zinn?
    A. Abducens nerve
    B. Inferior division of oculomotor nerve
    C. Superior division of oculomotor nerve
    D. Trochlear nerve

11) Which of the following extraocular muscles originate from the annulus of Zinn?
    A. Inferior oblique
    B. Medial rectus
    C. Superior oblique
    D. Levator palpebrae superioris

12) Which one of the following cranial nerve palsies results in a "down and out" appearance of the affected eye?
    A. Optic nerve
    B. Oculomotor nerve
    C. Trochlear nerve
    D. Abducens nerve

13) Which of the following is **FALSE** with regard to eyelid ptosis?
    A. Myasthenia gravis can result in a neurogenic ptosis
    B. The upper eyelid is lower in position in the affected eye
    C. Horner syndrome can result in a neurogenic ptosis
    D. Dermatochalasis can result in a mechanical ptosis

14) Which of the following is **NOT** a surgical correction technique for ptosis?
    A. Conjunctiva-Müller resection
    B. Levator advancement (resection)
    C. Lateral tarsal strip procedure
    D. Brow suspension

15) Which of the following is **FALSE** regarding an ectropion?
    A. Involutional ectropion typically affects the lower eyelid
    B. It can result in epiphora
    C. Facial nerve palsy can result in ectropion
    D. Opening the mouth can reduce the degree of eversion in cicatricial ectropion

16) Which of the following is **FALSE** regarding the Marcus Gunn jaw-winking syndrome?
   A. There is unilateral ptosis in the vast majority of reported cases
   B. The mandibular branch of the trigeminal nerve (V_3) aberrantly innervates the levator muscle
   C. Retraction of the ptotic eyelid following stimulation of the ipsilateral pterygoid muscle
   D. Jaw-winking improves with age

17) Which one of the following describes the correct relationship regarding the tear film layers?
   A. The glands of Krause contribute to the mucin layer
   B. The meibomian glands contribute to the mucin layer
   C. The glands of Manz contribute to the aqueous layer
   D. The glands of Wolfring contribute to the aqueous layer

18) Which of the following is **FALSE** regarding Lockwood's ligament?
   A. It prevents the downward displacement of the eyeball
   B. The inferior rectus muscle is enclosed within the ligament
   C. The inferior oblique muscle is not enclosed within the ligament
   D. Medial and lateral attachments of the ligament attach to the medial and lateral rectus sheaths

19) Which **TWO** of the following are **CORRECT** yoke muscle pairings?
   A. Superior rectus and inferior oblique
   B. Inferior rectus and medial rectus
   C. Inferior rectus and superior oblique
   D. Superior rectus and lateral rectus

20) Which of the following structures prevents the backflow of tears into the canaliculi from the lacrimal sac?
   A. Valve of Hasner
   B. Valve of Rosenmüller
   C. Valve of Hasner and the valve of Rosenmüller
   D. Valve of Krause

21) Which one of the following correctly depicts the flow of tears in the lacrimal drainage system?
    A. Lacrimal gland → canaliculi → puncta → valve of Rosenmüller → nasolacrimal sac → nasolacrimal duct → valve of Hasner
    B. Lacrimal gland → puncta → canaliculi → valve of Rosenmüller → nasolacrimal sac → valve of Hasner → nasolacrimal duct
    C. Lacrimal gland → puncta → canaliculi → valve of Rosenmüller → valve of Hasner → nasolacrimal sac → nasolacrimal duct
    D. Lacrimal gland → puncta → canaliculi → valve of Rosenmüller → nasolacrimal sac → nasolacrimal duct → valve of Hasner

22) Which of the following is **TRUE** regarding blepharitis?
    A. Anterior blepharitis is usually caused by meibomian gland dysfunction or pathology in gland secretions
    B. *Streptococcus pyogenes* is a common causative pathogen in chronic blepharitis
    C. Seborrheic blepharitis is strongly associated with generalised atopic dermatitis
    D. Staphylococcal blepharitis is associated with atopic dermatitis

23) Which of the following is **FALSE** regarding lacrimal irrigation?
    A. Lacrimal irrigation is contraindicated in acute dacryocystitis
    B. A "hard stop" and no saline efflux into the throat indicates a nasolacrimal duct obstruction
    C. A "soft stop" indicates a nasolacrimal duct obstruction
    D. Nasolacrimal duct obstruction may result in the reflux of purulent material

24) Which of the following is **TRUE** regarding nasolacrimal system pathology?
    A. Dacryolithiasis often presents early in childhood and is more common in females
    B. Neonatal nasolacrimal duct obstruction requires urgent intervention within the first year of life
    C. *Actinomyces israelii* is a common causative pathogen for chronic canaliculitis
    D. Chronic dacryoscystitis rarely presents with epiphora

25) Which of the following is more commonly seen in children?
    A. Capillary haemangioma
    B. Cavernous haemangioma
    C. Pleomorphic lacrimal gland adenoma
    D. Optic nerve meningioma

Chapter 7

Ocular Adnexal and Orbital Disease Answers

1) C
The lesser wing of the sphenoid is part of the roof of the orbit. The orbital floor is comprised of three bones: the maxilla, zygoma and palatine. Of clinical significance is the relative weakness of the posterior and medial aspects of the maxillary bone, which renders it susceptible to "blowout" fractures in trauma.

2) D
The frontal bone and the lesser wing of the sphenoid are the two bones that comprise the roof of the orbit. The medial wall meanwhile consists of 4 bones: the maxilla, lacrimal, ethmoid and sphenoid.

3) C
The superior orbital fissure transmits CN III, CN IV and CN VI as well as the first division of the CN V, which has already divided into the nasociliary, frontal and lacrimal branches. The relationship between these structures and the annulus of Zinn (the common origin of the four recti muscles) is shown in the figure below.

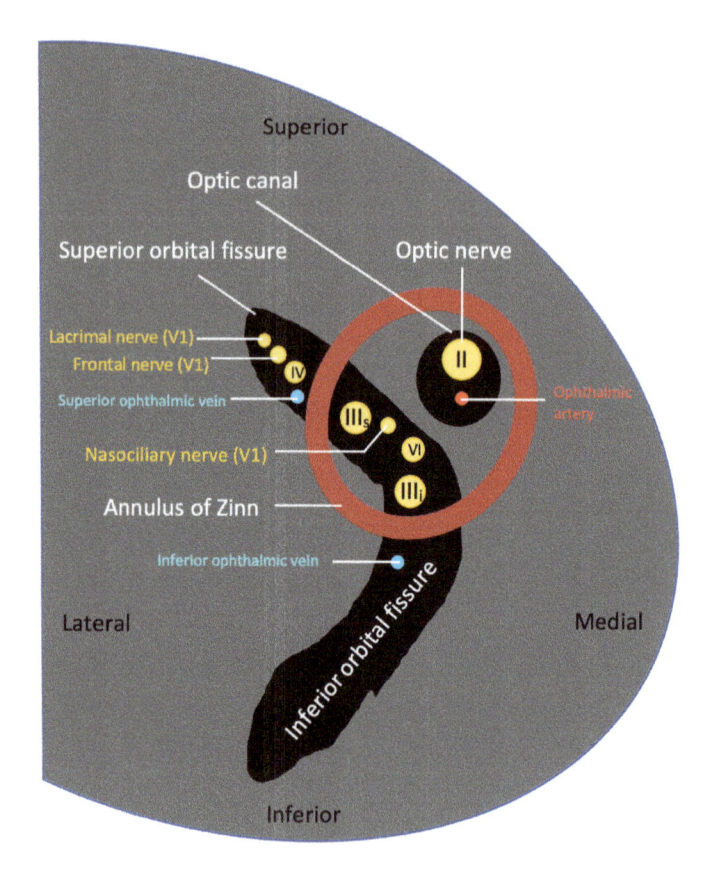

[Diagram of right orbital apex showing: Superior, Optic canal, Optic nerve, Superior orbital fissure, Lacrimal nerve (V1), Frontal nerve (V1), Superior ophthalmic vein, Nasociliary nerve (V1), Annulus of Zinn, Inferior ophthalmic vein, Inferior orbital fissure, Ophthalmic artery, with cranial nerves II, III, IV, VI labelled; Lateral, Medial, Inferior orientations marked]

Tolosa-Hunt syndrome refers to a rare, idiopathic inflammation of this fissure, which results in a number of clinical signs.

4) B
Proptosis refers to the displacement of any organ or body part but is commonly used to refer to the eyes. Axial proptosis sees the forward displacement of the globe in the axial plane and is typically the result of retrobulbar lesions or space-occupying lesions within the muscle cone. Bilateral proptosis is most commonly caused by thyroid eye disease. This is often referred to as exophthalmos.

Dystopia refers to the displacement of the globe in the coronal plane, resulting in a malalignment of both eyes in the horizontal plane. This type of displacement is often due to extraconal mass lesions such as lacrimal gland tumours.

Superior displacement can be caused by tumours from the maxillary sinus invading upwards through the floor of the orbit.

5) D

In a forced duction test, the patient is administered topical anaesthesia, and using forceps, the insertion point of the muscles in the affected eye is grasped, and the globe rotated in the direction of reduced mobility. In a neurological deficit, no resistance is encountered.

A differential intraocular pressure (IOP) test first measures the IOP at rest, while movement is not attempted. Then, with the patient attempting to move the eye in the direction of reduced mobility, the IOP is remeasured. In muscle restrictive ophthalmoplegia, an increase of >6 mmHg is seen.

Saccadic eye movements refer to the patient rapidly and swiftly moving both eyes between two fixed points in the same plane. Neurological ophthalmoplegia would result in a reduced velocity whereas restrictive lesions would result in normal velocity followed by a restriction in movement beyond a certain point.

6) D

Phthisis bulbi refers to a small, shrunken and non-functional eye that may result from severe ocular disease or trauma.

Optic neuropathy is a serious and potentially sight-threatening complication of thyroid eye disease (TED). Swollen orbital tissues and enlarged recti muscles secondary to TED can result in compression of the optic nerve and restriction in its blood flow.

Lid retraction occurs in about 50% of those with Graves disease. As a result, patients may report difficulty in blinking and a "staring" appearance. The Kocher sign describes this staring appearance, which is particularly marked on attentive fixation.

Thirty to 50 percent of patients with TED will also develop ophthalmoplegia secondary to a restrictive myopathy. This is a result of oedema and fibrosis of the extraocular muscles secondary to inflammation.

7) D

Streptococcus pneumoniae, Staphylococcus aureus and *Streptococcus pyogenes* are all common causes of bacterial orbital cellulitis. *Haemophilus influenzae* is also a common cause, especially in children. Orbital cellulitis usually results from a spread of injection from the adjacent paranasal sinuses. It can also arise from preseptal cellulitis, trauma, ocular surgery or even dental infection.

Patients typically present with a sudden, rapidly progressive painful red eye that is made worse by eye movements. There is also often marked pyrexia with tender, firm eyelids. There may be a recent history of respiratory or sinus symptoms.

8) C
Carotid-cavernous sinus fistulae are a result of an arteriovenous fistula between the carotid artery and cavernous sinus. These shunts result in ocular manifestations owing to the following mechanisms:

- Reduced blood flow to the cranial nerves
- Increased episcleral venous pressure
- Venous and arterial stasis around the orbit

Trauma is the most common (75%) cause of direct shunts and patients usually present days or weeks following a head injury with a triad of pulsatile proptosis, conjunctival chemosis and with reports of hearing a whooshing noise.

In most cases these fistulae are not life threatening and surgery is only indicated if there is no spontaneous resolution of the fistulae. Indirect carotid-cavernous fistulae have the shunt via the meningeal arteries and often close spontaneously.

9) B
Dacryops is often a bilateral cyst originating from the lacrimal gland, which develops secondary to an obstructed, dilated lacrimal duct. It arises from the palpebral lobe of the lacrimal gland and protrudes into the superior fornix.

10) D
The annulus of Zinn is a tendinous ring at the apex of the orbit, from which 6 important structures pass (see figure in answer to Question 3):

- Superior division of the oculomotor nerve
- Inferior division of the oculomotor nerve
- Abducens nerve
- Nasociliary branch of the ophthalmic division of trigeminal nerve (V_1)
- Optic nerve
- Ophthalmic artery

The trochlear nerve emerges from the superior orbital fissure outside the annulus of Zinn.

Ocular Adnexal and Orbital Disease Answers

11) B

There are 7 extraocular muscles located in the orbit that control the movement of the eyeball and eyelid. The 4 recti muscles (superior rectus, inferior rectus, medial rectus and lateral rectus) all originate from the annulus of Zinn and pass anteriorly to insert on the sclera.

The superior and inferior oblique originate from the sphenoid bone and orbital floor, respectively. The levator palpebrae superioris originates from the sphenoid bone and attaches to the tarsal plate of the eyelid.

12) B

An optic nerve palsy would be a sensory palsy resulting in visual impairment.

The oculomotor nerve innervates all extraocular muscles except for the lateral rectus and superior oblique. Unopposed action of the superior oblique and lateral rectus muscles in CN III palsy results in depression and abduction ("down and out" appearance) of the eyeball.

Abducens nerve palsy will result in an abduction deficit and a deviation worse in the direction of the palsy.

13) A

Eyelid ptosis manifests itself with the upper eyelid resting abnormally low. Ptosis can be classified by its aetiology. Neurogenic ptosis can be caused by CN III palsy or Horner syndrome. Myogenic ptosis includes myopathies of the levator palpebrae superioris or neuromuscular junction abnormalities such as myasthenia gravis and myotonic dystrophy. Dermatochalasis (overhanging skin on the eyelid) can be mistaken for ptosis. However, it can also result in mechanical ptosis.

14) C

The common surgical techniques for lid ptosis correction include:

- **Conjunctiva-Müller resection**: the Müller muscle is excised along with overlying conjunctiva and the resected edges are reattached. This is usually performed in cases of mild ptosis (e.g., Horner syndrome)
- **Levator advancement (resection)**: the levator is shortened by either an anterior or posterior approach. The extent of resection is determined by the degree of preoperative ptosis
- **Brow suspension**: Typically used in cases of severe ptosis where there is poor levator function, for instance, in cases of 3rd nerve

palsies. A prolene/silicone/autologous fascia sling is used to suspend the tarsal plate from the frontalis muscle.

A lateral tarsal strip procedure is used to repair generalised ectropion.

15) D

Age-related (involutional) ectropion typically affects the lower eyelid manifesting as an eversion of the eyelid. This can result in epiphora (tear overflow). Facial nerve palsy results in an ipsilateral paralytic ectropion. There may be retraction of both the upper and lower eyelids as well as brow ptosis. Cicatricial ectropion is caused by scarring or fibrosis that subsequently pulls the eyelid away. Opening the mouth will often **exacerbate** the ectropion.

16) D

The Marcus Gunn jaw-winking syndrome is a type of congenital neurogenic ptosis. In the majority of cases, there is unilateral ptosis. Upon stimulation of the ipsilateral pterygoid muscle, the ptotic eyelid is rapidly retracted. The stimulation can be in the form of chewing, sucking or opening the mouth. The exact aetiology is unclear, but it is believed to be caused by an aberrant innervation of the levator muscle by the mandibular branch of the trigeminal nerve (CN V_3). Jaw-winking does not improve with age.

17) D

The tear film is comprised of three layers: mucin, aqueous and lipid layer. Different glands contribute to each layer as follows:

- **Mucin layer**
  - Goblet cells
  - Glands of Manz
  - Crypts of Henle
- **Aqueous layer**
  - Glands of Krause
  - Glands of Wolfring
  - Lacrimal gland
- **Lipid layer**
  - Meibomian glands

Ocular Adnexal and Orbital Disease Answers

18) C
Often compared to a hammock due to its function, Lockwood's ligament has a suspensory role, preventing the downward displacement of the eye. It encloses both the inferior rectus and inferior oblique muscles. It extends laterally and medially to attach to the sheaths of the lateral and medial recti muscles, thereby forming an indirect attachment to the orbit.

19) A & C
Yoke muscles refer to muscle pairs that work in combination to achieve conjugate eye movements where the two eyes move together in the same direction. For instance, the left lateral rectus and right medial rectus work together to allow a left gaze.

20) B
There were many eponymous valves of the lacrimal system described in the early 20th century. However, modern imaging techniques have shown that many of these are not true valves, but rather, mucosal folds. Nonetheless, the valves of Rosemüller and Hasner are two eponymous valves that are still discussed and described in the present literature.

The valve of Rosenmüller, found at the junction of the lacrimal sac and common canaliculus, prevents the reflux of tears from the lacrimal sac into the common canaliculus. The valve of Hasner overlies the opening of the nasolacrimal duct into the inferior nasal meatus.

21) D
Tears from the orbital and palpebral lacrimal glands flow into the puncta that are located at the posterior edge of the medial lid margin. From there, tears flow in the canaliculi vertically before turning horizontally and medially to join the lacrimal sac. Within the junction between the common canaliculus and the lacrimal sac is the valve of Rosenmüller, which prevents reflux from the lacrimal sac to the puncta. From the lacrimal sac, tears flow into the nasolacrimal duct and into the inferior nasal meatus through the valve of Hasner.

22) D
Blepharitis can either be anterior and posterior, and it is useful to divide it as such, given that each has divergent aetiologies. In reality, there is usually a significant overlap between the two (mixed blepharitis).

- **Anterior**: can be seborrheic in origin where there is a strong link with generalised seborrheic dermatitis. *Staphylococcus aureus* is a common causative agent. There is also a strong association with atopic dermatitis.
- **Posterior**: caused by a dysfunction of the meibomian gland. It can be more persistent than its anterior counterpart and there is an association with acne roscea.

23) C

Lacrimal irrigation is usually performed in patients presenting with epiphora. It is, however, contraindicated if there is a concurrent infection of the nasolacrimal drainage system (i.e., acute dacryocystitis). On entering the lacrimal sac, a "hard stop" occurs as the tip of the blunt irrigation cannula meets the medial wall of the lacrimal sac, through which the rigid lacrimal bone can be felt. Gentle saline irrigation is then attempted. Following this, if the saline is tasted by the patient in their throat, then the lacrimal drainage system can be said to be patent. However, saline would not be tasted in cases of nasolacrimal duct obstruction and purulent material may be regurgitated. A "soft stop" indicates the presence of a canalicular obstruction. It is experienced if the cannula stops at or is proximal to the junction of the common canaliculus and the lacrimal sac. The sac is thus not entered — a spongy sensation ("soft stop") is felt, as the cannula presses against the soft tissue of the common canaliculus and the lateral wall of the lacrimal sac.

24) C

Dacryolithiasis refers to the presence of lacrimal stones within the nasolacrimal drainage system. Patients often present in late adulthood with reports of intermittent epiphora and recurrent infections. Dacryolithiasis is more common in females. Nasolacrimal duct obstruction is seen in approximately 5% of neonates and spontaneous resolution occurs in the majority (85%) within the first year of life.

Chronic canaliculitis is a relatively uncommon condition that is frequently caused by *Actinomyces israelii* (Gram positive rod). Patients often present with unilateral epiphora, a pouting punctum and yellow mucopurulent discharge. Chronic dacryocystitis often presents with chronic epiphora, which may be associated with recurrent or chronic conjunctivitis.

25) A

Capillary haemangioma (strawberry naevus) is the second most common benign orbital tumour in children (after dermoid cyst). The majority (80%) of lesions resolve by the age of 8 and treatment (e.g., beta-blockers) is only indicated if they cause visual impairment. Optic nerve meningioma, cavernous haemangioma and pleomorphic lacrimal gland adenoma are typically seen in middle-aged adults.

Chapter 8: Refractive Errors and Optics Questions

1) What is the average dimension of the normal human adult eye?
   A. Globe: 24.2 mm (horizontal) × 23.7 mm (vertical), Cornea: 12 mm (horizontal) × 11.5 mm (vertical)
   B. Globe: 23.7 mm (horizontal) × 24.2 mm (vertical), Cornea: 12 mm (horizontal) × 11.5 mm (vertical)
   C. Globe: 23.7 mm (horizontal) × 24.2 mm (vertical), Cornea: 11.5 mm (horizontal) × 12 mm (vertical)
   D. Globe 24.2 mm (horizontal) × 23.7 mm (vertical), Cornea: 11.5 mm (horizontal) × 12 mm (vertical)

2) What colour ranges are the three colour-sensitive cones in the retina **MOST** sensitive to?
   A. Red, blue and yellow
   B. Red, green and blue
   C. Green, yellow and blue
   D. Green, yellow and red

3) John Doe suffers from a type of colour blindness where "green" cones (also known as M-cone) are missing. What is this type of colour blindness called?
   A. Tritanopia
   B. Achromatopia
   C. Protanopia
   D. Deuteranopia

4) Which of the following is **NOT** associated with a refractive error of +8.00D?
   A. Amblyopia
   B. Esotropia
   C. Buphthalmos
   D. Acute angle closure glaucoma

5) Which of the following test is used to examine visual acuity in children less than 4 months old?
   A. Bailey-Lovie chart
   B. Teller and Keeler cards
   C. Crowded Kay pictures
   D. Sonksen crowded tests

6) Which of the following is **FALSE** about intraocular lens power calculation formulae?
   A. The Haigis formula requires a measured anterior chamber depth (ACD)
   B. The Hoffer Q is preferable in eyes with shorter axial lengths (<22 mm)
   C. Third-generation formulae such as the SRK-T and Holladay 1 require a measured ACD
   D. The SRK-T formula is preferable in eyes with longer axial lengths (>26 mm)

7) Which of the following tests does **NOT** require binocular vision?
   A. Maddox rod
   B. Bagolini striated glasses
   C. Worth four-dot test
   D. Duochrome test

8) In LASIK (laser-assisted in situ keratomileusis) for myopia, which of the following is **TRUE**?
   A. There is flattening of the central cornea
   B. There is steepening of the central cornea
   C. There is flattening of the peripheral cornea
   D. There is steepening of the peripheral cornea

9) Which of the following is a low vision aid for distant objects?
   A. Newtonian telescope
   B. Loupes
   C. Galilean telescope
   D. Microscope

10) Which of the following criterion would qualify for a Group 2 (large lorries and buses) driving licence in the UK?
   A. Best corrected visual acuity of 6/9 (Snellen) in both eyes
   B. Ability to read a standard number plate from 19 m
   C. Patching of one eye
   D. Homonymous hemianopia

11) Which of the following is **NOT** a test to detect sensory fusion abnormality?
   A. Worth four-dot test
   B. Bagolini striated glasses
   C. Lang test
   D. 4 Δ prism test

12) Which of the following is **TRUE** regarding a prism dioptre?
   A. 1 prism dioptre is equal to 2 degrees
   B. 1 prism dioptre refracts a beam of light to a point at 1 m
   C. 1 prism dioptre refracts a beam of light 10 cm towards the apex at 1 m
   D. 1 prism dioptre refracts a beam of light 1 cm towards the base at 1 m

13) Which of the following is **TRUE** regarding logMAR charts?
   A. No perception of light gives a logMAR score of 1.0
   B. A logMAR score of 0.1 represents a better visual acuity compared to a score of −0.1
   C. Each letter is equal to a logMAR score of 0.02
   D. There are 6 letters per line

14) Which of the following is **MOST** commonly measured by optical coherence tomography?
   A. Photoreceptor function
   B. Retinal thickness
   C. Retinal ischaemia
   D. Corneal curvature

15) What is the refractive power of the cornea?
   A. 39D
   B. 43D
   C. 53D
   D. 59D

16) Which is of the following is **FALSE** about accommodation?
    A. The RAF rule is used to measure the amplitude of accommodation
    B. Cyclopentolate abolishes accommodation
    C. Usually starts to decline after the age of 50 years
    D. There is a strict relationship between accommodation and convergence

17) Which is of the following is **TRUE** about hypermetropia?
    A. Should be fully corrected in esotropic children
    B. Delays the onset of presbyopia
    C. Is present in 80% of children between the ages of 2 and 6 years
    D. Aphakia is a form of hypermetropia

18) The image formed by a thin concave lens is:
    A. Virtual, erect, diminished
    B. Virtual, erect, enlarged
    C. Real, erect, diminished
    D. Real, inverted, enlarged

19) A patient complains of decreased right vision (visual acuity: OD 6/36, OS 6/6). Full ocular examination is unremarkable, and a diagnosis of functional visual loss is suspected. Which of the following would be **MOST** useful in supporting this diagnosis?
    A. Optokinetic nystagmus (OKN) drum
    B. Cycloplegic refraction
    C. Mirror test
    D. Prism cover test

20) Which of the following colour vision status is **MOST** likely present in a patient with Wernicke encephalopathy?
    A. Total colour blindness
    B. Blue-yellow colour blindness
    C. Red-green colour blindness
    D. Normal colour vision

21) Which of the following is **NOT** a test for stereopsis?
    A. Krimsky test
    B. Titmus test
    C. Frisby test
    D. TNO test

22) Which of the following lenses is **MOST** appropriate in correcting a refractive error of +1.00 / −3.00 × 90°?
    A. Convex lens
    B. Concave lens
    C. Periscopic lens
    D. Toric lens

23) A 13-year-old boy reports recent difficulty over the past year in reading the board in front of his classroom. He has no issues with reading his books. A full ocular examination was unremarkable and an assessment with retinoscopy revealed significant refractive error. What is the **MOST** likely refractive error and appropriate type of lens to address this?
    A. Myopia and convex lens
    B. Hypermetropia and convex lens
    C. Myopia and concave lens
    D. Hypermetropia and concave lens

24) The following can be used for the correction of unilateral aphakia **EXCEPT**:
    A. Anterior chamber intraocular lens
    B. Glasses
    C. Posterior chamber intraocular lens
    D. Contact lens

25) The refractive state of the eye may be altered by the following **EXCEPT**:
    A. Vitreous humour removal
    B. Ciliary muscle paralysis
    C. Changing the anterior chamber depth
    D. Changing the axial length of the eye

Chapter 8

Refractive Errors and Optics Answers

1) A
The globe is generally less tall than it is wide. It grows rapidly, increasing from about 16–17 mm at birth to 22.5–23 mm by 3 years of age. By age 12, the eye attains its full size. Similar to the globe, the cornea is slightly wider horizontally than it is vertically.

2) B
A special property of the cone system is colour vision. Unlike rods, which contain a single photopigment, there are 3 types of cones that differ in the photopigment they contain. Each of these has a different sensitivity to light of different wavelengths, and for this reason are referred to as "blue", "green" and "red", or more appropriately, short-wavelength (S-cone), middle-wavelength (M-cone) and long-wavelength (L-cone), respectively, which describe their spectral sensitivities.

3) D
Deuteranopia (also called green-blind) is a type of colour blindness in which the middle-wavelength (M-cone; "green") cones are missing. Tritanopia and protanopia refer to the absence of short-wavelength (S-cone; "blue") and long-wavelength (L-cone; "red"), respectively. Protanopia and deuteranopia are hereditary and sex-linked, affecting predominantly males. Tritanopia, on the other hand, is related to chromosome 7 and is therefore not sex-linked. It can also be acquired rather than inherited. Achromatopia refers to total colour blindness, where there is an inability to perceive all colours.

4) C
Hypermetropia can be divided into low (≤ +2.00D), moderate (+2.25 to +5.00D) and high (> +5.00D). High hypermetropia is associated with refractive amblyopia, accommodative esotropia and acute angle closure glaucoma. Refractive amblyopia can develop in children with large

amounts of uncorrected hypermetropia. Hypermetropia that is not fully compensated with accommodation will force the eye into convergence with a resultant accommodative esotropia. Hypermetropic eyes are often shorter in axial length, which increases the risk of acute angle closure glaucoma. Microphthalmos and nanophthalmos (rather than buphthalmos) are associated with high hypermetropia.

5) B
Evaluation of vision in preverbal children (usually <2 years old) can be separated into the qualitative assessment of visual behaviour and the quantitative assessment of visual acuity, using preferential looking tests. The latter is based on the fact that infants prefer to look at a pattern rather than a homogenous stimulus. An example of this is the Teller and Keeler acuity cards, which consist of black stripes (gratings) of varying widths. The infant is exposed to this and the examiner observes the eyes for fixation movements.

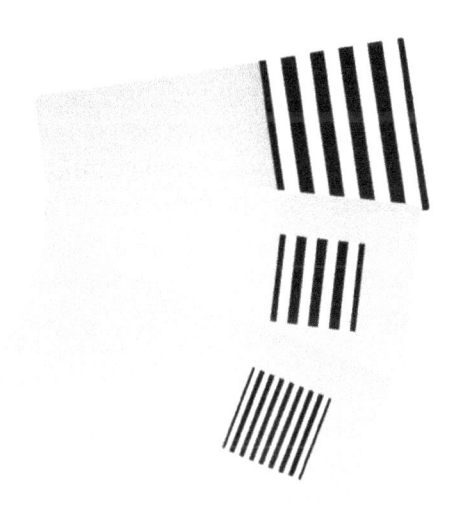

Teller acuity cards

The other options are used to test visual acuity in verbal children. Crowded Kay pictures are usually used in children aged 2 and above, as they will have sufficient language skills to undertake a picture-naming test. At 3 years of age, most children will be able to undertake the matching letter optotypes in crowded letter tests such as the Sonksen or Keeler logMAR crowded tests. Older children may continue with the crowded letter tests or proceed on to the standard logMAR chart.

6) C

Third-generation formulae such as the SRK-T and Holladay 1 are based only on two measurements (keratometry and axial length) as well as a single intraocular lens constant.

7) D

The duochrome test is commonly used to refine the best vision sphere during monocular refraction. Binocular vision is therefore not a prerequisite for the duochrome test. The other tests require functional binocular vision.

8) A

LASIK is a surgical procedure designed to correct refractive errors. It involves creating a corneal flap using a microkeratome, reshaping the cornea using an excimer laser to remove tissue from the underlying stromal bed and then replacing the flap.

LASIK, when used to correct myopia and myopic astigmatism, accomplishes this by ablating the central corneal tissue and flattening the central anterior corneal curvature. This reduces the dioptric power of the cornea and allows accurate correction of myopic defects.

On the other hand, LASIK accomplishes this by ablating an annular zone at the periphery of the cornea when used to correct hypermetropia and hypermetropic astigmatism. The desired refractive effect is achieved by causing relative flattening of the peripheral cornea and concomitantly relative steepening of the central cornea.

9) C

The Galilean telescope is an optical low-vision aid for distance. It consists of 2 lenses: (1) an objective lens (a convex lens closest to the object) and (2) an ocular lens (a concave lens closest to the eye). The image produced is real and erect.

The Newtonian telescope is used mainly in astronomy. The microscope and loupes are magnification devices used to view near, small objects in better detail.

10) B

In addition to the minimum standard requirement of the ability to read a standard number plate from 20 metres, Group 2 (bus and lorry drivers) driving licences in the UK require a higher standard of visual acuity. This includes visual acuity, with corrective lenses if necessary, of at least

Snellen 6/7.5 in the better eye and at least Snellen 6/60 in the worse eye. If lenses are used to attain these values, correction must be by glasses with power not exceeding +8 dioptres, or by contact lenses. Monocularity is not acceptable. The horizontal visual field with both eyes should be at least 160°, and no defects (e.g., homonymous hemianopia) should be present within a radius of the central 30°.

11) C

The Lang test is used to measure stereopsis rather than differentiate between the different sensory anomalies.

The Worth four-dot test and Bagolini striated glasses are tests for sensory anomalies and can be used to differentiate between binocular single vision (BSV), anomalous retinal correspondence (ARC) and suppression. Results can only be interpreted if the presence or absence of a manifest squint is known at the time of testing.

The 4 Δ prism test is another test for sensory fusion abnormality and is used to determine whether a patient has bifoveal fixation or a small central suppression scotoma (or foveal suppression).

12) D

The unit of measure of the prismatic displacement of an image is the prism dioptre [often abbreviated with the delta (Δ) symbol]:

- *A prism of 1 dioptre will produce a 1 cm visible displacement at 1 m*

As a general rule of thumb, the angle of deviation in degree is usually half of that of the corresponding prism dioptre. For example, a prism of 2 prism dioptre produces an angle of deviation of 1 degree.

A lens which incorporates prism correction will displace the viewed image horizontally, vertically or a combination of both directions. The most common application for this is the treatment of strabismus. By moving the image in front of the deviated eye, double vision can be avoided and a comfortable binocular vision achieved.

A prescription that specifies prism correction will specify the "base". Like a triangle, the base is the thickest part of the lens and is opposite from the apex, which is the thinnest edge. When a ray of light passes through a prism, it will be deviated towards the base. If you are looking through the prism, however, the image appears to be displaced toward the apex, because the image appears to originate from the direction of the deviated light ray (see figure below).

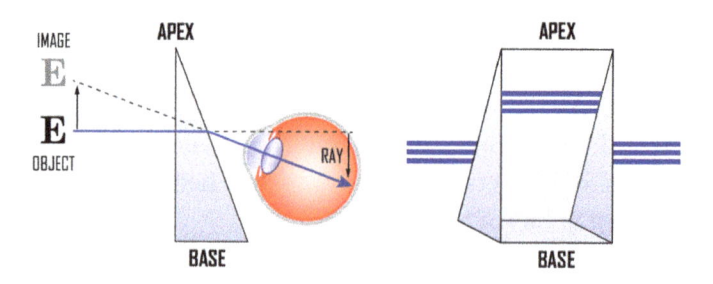

Deviation of light and resulting image in a prism

13) C

The logMAR charts present a series of 5 letters of equal difficulty on each row, with standardised spacing between letters and rows, for a total of 14 lines (and therefore a total of 70 letters).

In logMAR notation, lower scores (and therefore negative values) correspond to better vision, and as acuity becomes worse, the value of the logMAR increases. Each line on the chart represents a change of 0.1 log unit in the acuity level with each letter having a value of 0.02 log unit.

A logMAR score of 1.0 is equivalent to a Snellen acuity of 6/60. No perception of light is equivalent to a logMAR score of 3.0.

14) B

Optical coherence tomography (OCT) is an imaging technique that works similarly to an ultrasound. It uses light waves instead of sound waves. By using the time-delay information contained in the light waves that have been reflected from different structures inside the eye, the OCT system can reconstruct a depth-profile of these structures (e.g., retinal thickness).

Electroretinogram (ERG) testing is an important diagnostic tool for retinal and optic nerve pathology by measuring the function of rod and cone photoreceptors.

Fluorescein angiography is a technique for examining the circulation of the retina and choroid using a fluorescent dye and a specialised camera. Areas of non-perfusion often reflect the extent of retina involved due to ischaemia in diseases such as diabetic retinopathy.

Measurement of corneal curvature/power can be performed with a variety of instruments, most commonly, a keratometer or corneal topography device. Corneal curvature measurements are usually used for intraocular lens calculations and corneal refractive surgery. It is also helpful for contact lens fitting and detection of irregular astigmatism.

15) B

The cornea and the lens are the two main refractive elements of the human eye. The average optic power of the human eye is 60D, of which the cornea accounts for approximately two thirds (43D) and the lens one third (17D). While the cornea contributes most of the eye's refractive power, its focus is fixed, unlike the lens where its refractive power can be changed via the process of accommodation.

16) C

Presbyopia is the gradual loss of the eyes' accommodative ability to focus on near objects. The onset of this is usually shortly after the age of 40 years.

The ciliary muscle is predominantly under the control of the parasympathetic nervous system, and antimuscarinic drugs such as atropine and cyclopentolate temporarily paralyse the ciliary muscle, abolishing accommodation.

The relationship between accommodation and convergence is a tight, linear one. For each impulse of change in accommodation, there is a corresponding impulse of change in convergence. This occurs in a consistent ratio known as the AC (accommodative convergence)/A (accommodation) ratio.

The RAF rule provides an objective measurement of the amplitude of accommodation.

17) D

Aphakia is the absence of the crystalline lens either due to congenital or acquired (e.g., cataract surgery) causes. There is high hypermetropia in aphakia with marked defective vision for both near and far distances.

Esotropia in children can be due to a variety of causes and is broadly classified into accommodative and non-accommodative types. The former refers to esotropia caused by the accommodative efforts in response to a hypermetropic refractive error. The initial treatment for this is the correction of the existing refractive error. Treatment for other causes of esotropia (i.e., non-accommodative type) will depend on the underlying aetiology.

Hypermetropia is known to be associated with early, rather than late, onset presbyopia.

The overall prevalence of hypermetropia is around 10%. Most full-term infants are mildly hypermetropic and the prevalence of hypermetropia in children is <10% (ranging from 8.4% at 6 years of age to approximately 1% at the age of 15 years).

18) A
The image formed by a thin concave lens will always be virtual, erect and diminished.

19) B
The OKN drum and mirror test are useful in detecting gross vision when the patient claims to be blind (i.e., visual acuity of hand movement, perception of light and no perception of light). These tests are not sensitive enough to diagnose milder factitious visual deficit (i.e., visual acuity of 6/36 in our case) for which cycloplegic refraction is useful in discovering any uncorrected refractive errors.

The prism cover test measures the angle of deviation for near and/or distance fixation and has no role in the diagnosis of functional visual loss.

20) C
As a general rule of thumb: blue-yellow defects tend to be produced by macular diseases (e.g., age-related macular degeneration), whereas red-green defects are usually a result of optic nerve disorders (e.g., optic neuritis, optic atrophy, tobacco-alcohol optic neuropathy). There is often a history of excessive alcohol consumption in Wernicke encephalopathy, which would give rise to tobacco-alcohol optic neuropathy.

21) A
The Krimsky test is used to quantify ocular deviation by determining how much prism is required to centre the corneal reflex.

22) D
A refractive error is expressed by the spectacle (or contact lens) prescription required to correct it in the form: sphere/cylinder X angle of the cylinder axis.

Sphere indicates the amount of lens power, measured in dioptres, prescribed to correct myopia or hypermetropia. If the number for this is negative, it implies myopia (and vice versa). If there is only a sphere prescription, it means that the correction for myopia or hypermetropia is "spherical", or equal in all meridians of the eye. In such a case, a simple convex (+ve) or concave (-ve) lens will be required for the correction of hypermetropia or myopia, respectively.

Cylinder indicates the amount of lens power for astigmatism. If there is no cylinder prescription, it means that there is no astigmatism that requires correction. The term "cylinder" means that the lens power added to correct astigmatism is not spherical, but instead toric. A toric lens is a lens with different optical power and focal length in two orientations perpendicular to each other. Such a lens behaves like a combination of a spherical lens and a cylindrical lens. Similar to spherical prescription, the number for cylinder prescription may be negative (in which case it will be for the correction of myopic astigmatism) or positive (for the correction of hypermetropic astigmatism).

Periscopic lenses are mainly used in photography and give good definition of the peripheral visual field.

23) C

Myopia (short-sightedness) is a common refractive error where affected individuals are unable to see clearly in the distance. It occurs when the shape of the eye causes light rays to bend (refract) incorrectly, focusing the resulting image in front of the retina. Concave (minus) lenses are required to correct myopic refractive error.

24) B

Glasses correction in unilateral aphakia poses a barrier to binocular vision due to aniseikonia (difference in retinal image size between the two eyes) and large prismatic effects encountered in the peripheral portion of the lens. The former causes significant magnification difference to the point where binocular single vision is impossible.

Contact lens fitted on the aphakic eye gives the advantage of fusion (i.e., the use of both eyes together). It also has the cosmetic benefit of giving the aphakic eye a completely normal appearance, instead of the need for thick, heavy glasses.

The insertion of an intraocular lens (either anterior chamber or posterior chamber) is routinely performed during cataract surgery, in which the patient's cataract is removed and replaced with an artificial intraocular lens.

25) A

The vitreous is made up of 99% water. Its refractive index is 1.336, which is identical to that of the aqueous. Removal of the vitreous alone does not alter the refractive status unless the vitreous chamber is filled with silicone oil or gas.

The ciliary muscle is involved in the process of accommodation. Paralysing the ciliary muscle will result in a loss of accommodation with a subsequent reduction in the plus power of the lens (i.e., the patient will become less myopic/more hypermetropic).

Changing the depth of the anterior chamber will alter the effectivity of the lens and hence the refractive power.

The axial length of the eye is one of the main factors that determine the ocular refractive power. A shorter axial length results in hypermetropia and vice versa.

Mock Exam Paper Questions

1) A 48-year-old man with a history of asthma is seen in clinic with progressive visual deterioration. On fundoscopy, pallor of the optic disc is noted, along with bayonetting of the vessels around the cup. Automated perimetry shows nasal scotomata. Which of the following pharmacological agents would **NOT** be recommended for the management of this patient's condition?
   A. Timolol
   B. Brimonidine
   C. Acetazolamide
   D. Latanoprost

2) A patient with low vision uses a 16D lens as a simple magnifying glass. What is the **MOST** likely resultant magnification?
   A. 2x
   B. 5x
   C. 8x
   D. 11x

3) A 5-year-old girl is diagnosed with a moderate angled right esotropia. What is the **MOST** appropriate first step in treatment?
   A. Cycloplegic refraction
   B. Patching of the left eye
   C. Right medical rectus recession
   D. Observation

4) A 37-year-old female reports recent onset diplopia in primary position. On right gaze, there is reduced adduction of the left eye, which does not improve on covering the other eye. Vertical movements are normal. What is the **MOST** likely diagnosis?
   A. Consecutive exotropia
   B. Traumatic entrapment of left lateral rectus
   C. Duane syndrome
   D. Right internuclear ophthalmoplegia

5) Which of the following agents is typically **NOT** used for the initial treatment of acute angle-closure glaucoma?
   A. Topical latanoprost
   B. Topical dexamethasone
   C. Intravenous/oral acetazolamide
   D. Topical timolol

6) A patient has a spectacle correction of −1.50 / +3.00 × 90° for his right eye. Which of the following describes the optical characteristics of this patient's eye?
   A. −1.50 / +3.00 × 90°
   B. +3.00 / −1.50 × 90°
   C. −3.00 / +1.50 × 180°
   D. +1.50 / −3.00 × 180°

7) Which of the following modalities is used to measure corneal thickness?
   A. Ultrasonic pachymetry
   B. Fluorescein angiography
   C. Goldmann applanation tonometry
   D. Gonioscopy

8) Which of the following symptoms is a **commonly** noted side effect associated with prostaglandin analogues such as latanoprost?
   A. Reduction in vision in patients with pre-existing cataracts
   B. Loss of eyelashes
   C. Weight gain
   D. Increase in iris pigmentation

9) A 37-year-old man presents with an insidious onset of vertical diplopia. On alternate cover testing, there is evidence of left hypertropia, worse on left head tilt and right gaze. Which of the following muscle palsy is **MOST** likely to explain his symptoms?
   A. Left inferior rectus
   B. Left inferior oblique
   C. Right superior rectus
   D. Left superior oblique

10) A 12-year-old boy has been referred by his local optometrist for an incidental finding of elevated optic discs. On B-scan ultrasonography, there are hyperechoic lesions at the optic disc. What is the **MOST** likely diagnosis?
    A. Optic disc drusen
    B. Papilloedema
    C. Myelinated nerve fibres
    D. Optic disc coloboma

11) A 3-month-old girl has a growing red lesion on her right upper lid with associated ptosis. Her parents note that the lesion increases in size whenever she cries. What is the **MOST** likely diagnosis?
    A. Pyogenic granuloma
    B. Cavernous haemangioma
    C. Neurofibroma
    D. Capillary haemangioma

12) Which of the following statements regarding commonly used systemic drugs and their associated ocular side effects is **FALSE**?
    A. Amiodarone can cause abnormal colour vision
    B. Digoxin can lead to corneal deposits, described as vortex keratopathy
    C. Corticosteroids are associated with an increased risk of cataracts and glaucoma
    D. Vigabatrin can cause visual field defects

13) The following can be used in colour vision testing **EXCEPT**:
    A. Ishihara test
    B. Farnsworth-Munsell 100-hue test
    C. Watzke-Allen test
    D. Hardy-Rand-Rittler test

14) A 1-year-old boy presents with a squint and bilateral absence of red reflex. There is a family history of similar eye problems. What is the **MOST** likely diagnosis?
    A. Persistent fetal vasculature
    B. Retinoblastoma
    C. Coats disease
    D. Retinopathy of prematurity

15) A 2-month-old girl has a well-demarcated pink patch around the skin of her left eye, which does not blanch with pressure. She has recently been diagnosed with epilepsy. What is the **MOST** likely diagnosis?
    A. Sturge-Weber syndrome
    B. Von Hippel-Lindau syndrome
    C. Tuberous sclerosis
    D. Von Recklinghausen disease

16) A 4-month-old baby girl is not making any eye contact. On further questioning, the baby's mother mentions there was a history of maternal diabetes and excessive alcohol consumption during her pregnancy. What is the **MOST** likely diagnosis?
    A. Leber hereditary optic neuropathy
    B. Optic nerve hypoplasia
    C. Central serous chorioretinopathy
    D. Nutritional optic neuropathy

17) Which of the following is **TRUE** regarding the image formed by a prism?
    A. Erect, real, deviated towards the base
    B. Erect, virtual, deviated towards the apex
    C. Erect, real, deviated towards the apex
    D. Erect, virtual, deviated towards the base

18) Which of the following investigations provides the highest diagnostic yield in infective endophthalmitis?
    A. Anterior chamber tap
    B. Serology
    C. Vitreous biopsy
    D. Corneal scrape

19) Which of the following is **NOT** a common cause of gradual visual loss?
    A. Dry age-related macular degeneration
    B. Diabetic maculopathy
    C. Cataract
    D. Central retinal vein occlusion

20) A patient has regular astigmatism with a spectacle prescription of +1.00 / −2.50 × 90° in both eyes. She decides to correct this refractive error using toric contact lenses. Which of the following is **FALSE** about toric lenses?
    A. It has two meridians of curvature
    B. It has no power along its axis
    C. It forms a focal line parallel to its axis
    D. It is cylindrical in nature

21) Which of the following is the transposition equivalent of −2.00 / +1.00 × 120°?
    A. −3.00 / +1.00 × 120°
    B. −2.00 / −1.00 × 30°
    C. −1.00 / −1.00 × 30°
    D. +2.00 / −1.00 × 120°

22) Which of the following conditions is **unlikely** to present with a red eye?
    A. Acute anterior uveitis
    B. Acute angle-closure glaucoma
    C. Age-related macular degeneration
    D. Episcleritis

23) A 35-year-old Caucasian female presents with recurrent optic neuritis. An MRI brain shows characteristic periventricular white matter lesions. Which of the following medical therapy is **LEAST** likely to be indicated in the long-term management of her underlying condition?
    A. Interferon beta
    B. Natalizumab
    C. Methotrexate
    D. Glatiramer acetate

24) The following characteristic of a lens can be measured by a focimeter **EXCEPT**:
    A. Cylinder axis
    B. Prism power
    C. Optical centre
    D. Refractive index

25) Which of the following is **FALSE** about myopia?
    A. The second principal focus is in front of the retina
    B. Can be induced by central serous chorioretinopathy
    C. Can be induced by nucleosclerotic changes of the lens
    D. Can be treated with clear lens extraction

26) Which of the following is **FALSE** about the image formed by an indirect ophthalmoscope?
    A. Vertically inverted
    B. Horizontally inverted
    C. Relatively affected by the refractive state of the patient compared to direct ophthalmoscopy
    D. Real

27) A 75-year-old male presents with reduced right vision following uneventful cataract surgery in this eye 6 months ago. On examination, a white posterior capsular plaque and a low-grade anterior uveitis and vitritis are noted in his right eye. A diagnosis of delayed-onset postoperative endophthalmitis is suspected. What is the most likely causative organism?
    A. *Candida albicans*
    B. *Propionibacterium acnes*
    C. *Staphylococcus epidermidis*
    D. *Escherichia coli*

28) Which of the following is most likely responsible for vision in a patient with achromatopsia?
    A. Green cone cells
    B. Red cone cells
    C. Rod cells
    D. Bipolar cells

29) What does the acronym LASER stand for?
   A. Light Absorption by Stimulated Emission of Radiation
   B. Light Amplification by Stimulated Emission of Radiation
   C. Light Absorption by Synchronised Emission of Radiation
   D. Light Amplification by Synchronised Emission of Radiation

30) Which is the imaging modality of choice for a suspected intraocular foreign body?
   A. X-ray
   B. MRI
   C. CT
   D. Ultrasound

31) Which of the following is **FALSE** about atropine?
   A. The onset of cycloplegia usually precedes that of mydriasis
   B. It is a muscarinic antagonist
   C. Its mydriatic effect usually lasts longer than its cycloplegic effect
   D. It has a longer duration of action compared to cyclopentolate

32) Which of the following is **NOT** a metabolic cause for cataracts?
   A. Galactosaemia
   B. Hypoglycaemia
   C. Hypercalcaemia
   D. Hypoparathyroidism

33) Which of the following statements is TRUE regarding the human lens?
   A. It is made up of alpha, beta, delta and epsilon crystalline proteins
   B. Lens fibres do not have a nucleus or mitochondria
   C. There is an inverted Y suture in the anterior lens
   D. The posterior capsule becomes denser with age

34) Which of the following laser is used for capsulotomy?
   A. Nd:YAG laser
   B. Carbon dioxide laser
   C. Diode laser
   D. Excimer laser

35) Which of the following is the **MOST** likely cause for night vision loss in a 17-year-old boy?
   A. Best disease
   B. Cone dystrophy
   C. Cone-rod dystrophy
   D. Stargardt disease

36) All of the waves listed below are part of the electromagnetic spectrum **EXCEPT**:
   A. X-rays
   B. Sound waves
   C. Gamma rays
   D. Radio waves

37) When light passes from air into glass, its angle of refraction is:
   A. More than its angle of incidence
   B. Same as its angle of incidence
   C. Can be more or less than its angle of incidence
   D. Less than its angle of incidence

38) Which characteristic of light determines colour?
   A. Frequency
   B. Wavelength
   C. Neither of these
   D. Both of these

39) Which of the following is **NOT** a property of laser?
   A. It is polychromatic
   B. The waves of light are parallel
   C. All its photons have the same wavelength, which are in phase
   D. The distance between the mirrors within a laser tube is a multiple of the wavelength of the light emitted

40) Which of the following is **FALSE** about monovision?
   A. May reduce visual acuity
   B. Requires one eye to be made hypermetropic and the other myopic
   C. May reduce stereopsis
   D. Is mainly reserved for presbyopic patients

41) Which of the following is **FALSE** about the slit lamp?
    A. Cannot be used to examine the fundus
    B. Is a low-powered binocular compound microscope
    C. Contains prisms that shorten and invert the image
    D. Offers a stereoscopic view

42) Which of the following is **FALSE** about standard optical coherence tomography (OCT)?
    A. Uses reflection of infrared light to obtain retinal image
    B. Can detect subtle macular oedema
    C. Provides information on the circulation in the retina and choroid
    D. Provides resolution as small as 10 micrometres

43) Which of the following prescription has oblique astigmatism?
    A. $+2.00 / -2.50 \times 90°$
    B. $-3.00 / +1.00 \times 120°$
    C. $+1.00 / -1.00 \times 175°$
    D. $-4.00 / +3.00 \times 180°$

44) Which of the following is **TRUE** about the human crystalline lens?
    A. Contributes more refractive power than the cornea
    B. Has a uniform refractive index
    C. Has a longer radius of curvature anteriorly than posteriorly
    D. Has a refractive power of +25D

45) The following is true about contact lenses when compared with spectacles **EXCEPT**:
    A. Increases field of vision
    B. Reduces aniseikonia
    C. Reduces optical aberration
    D. Minify images in myopia

46) A 5-year-old boy presents with multiple brown organisms attached to the base of his eyelashes. There is a suspicion of sexual abuse. Which of the following is the **MOST** likely organism?
    A. *Phthirus pubis*
    B. *Pediculosis capitis*
    C. *Demodex folliculorum*
    D. *Borrelia burgdorferi*

47) Which of the following is the **MOST** common cause of bacterial conjunctivitis in children?
   A. *Moraxella catarrhalis*
   B. *Haemophilus influenzae*
   C. *Staphylococcus aureus*
   D. *Streptococcus pneumoniae*

48) Retinitis pigmentosa has the **WORST** prognosis when the mode of inheritance is:
   A. Autosomal dominant
   B. Autosomal recessive
   C. X-linked recessive
   D. Non-Mendelian

49) The **MOST** common congenital infection is
   A. Rubella
   B. Toxoplasmosis
   C. Herpes simplex virus
   D. Cytomegalovirus

50) A 10-year-old girl presents with bilateral blurry vision. Slit lamp examination revealed marked cells in the anterior chamber consistent with bilateral anterior uveitis. Which of the following is the **MOST** likely associated systemic condition?
   A. Juvenile idiopathic arthritis
   B. Sarcoidosis
   C. Tuberculosis
   D. Inflammatory bowel disease

51) A 3-month-old boy presents with epiphora and slight mucous discharge from the inferior punctum. He is systemically well. What is the **MOST** appropriate management?
   A. Punctal dilation and irrigation
   B. Hot compresses and gentle massage
   C. Punctal dilation and probing
   D. Topical antibiotic ointment

52) Which of the following does **NOT** pass through the superior orbital fissure?
    A. Optic nerve
    B. Oculomotor nerve
    C. Trochlear nerve
    D. Abducens nerve

53) Which of the following is **NOT** used in the measurement of the angle of deviation in strabismus?
    A. Hirschberg test
    B. Krimsky test
    C. Prism cover test
    D. Lang test

54) A 22-year-old male presents with difficulty opening both eyes, which he first noticed as a child. Clinical examination revealed severe bilateral ptosis and restriction of extraocular movements. A diagnosis of chronic progressive external ophthalmoplegia is made. Which of the following is **NOT** associated with this condition?
    A. Kearns-Sayre syndrome
    B. Parinaud syndrome
    C. Myotonic dystrophy
    D. Oculopharyngeal dystrophy

55) Which of the following is the **MOST** common location for an orbital blowout fracture?
    A. Orbital floor
    B. Medial orbital wall
    C. Lateral orbital wall
    D. Orbital roof

56) Which of the following rectus muscle inserts **closest** to the limbus?
    A. Inferior rectus
    B. Lateral rectus
    C. Medial rectus
    D. Superior rectus

57) Which of the following laser refractive techniques involves creation of a flap of the cornea?
   A. LASEK
   B. LASIK
   C. PRK
   D. Small incision lenticule extraction

58) Which of the following is NOT a treatment for seborrheic blepharitis?
   A. Eyelid scrubbing
   B. Oral azithromycin
   C. Oral flaxseed oil
   D. Oral lutein

59) A 43-year-old man has right corneal exposure. On further examination, he has paralysis of his right facial muscles including his forehead. He reports increased noise sensitivity and altered taste affecting the right side of his tongue. Where is the lesion?
   A. Brainstem
   B. Cerebellopontine angle
   C. Geniculate ganglion
   D. Stylomastoid foramen

60) A 5-year-old boy has mild cognitive impairment, upslanting palpebral fissures and large epicanthic folds. Which of the following is NOT a known ocular feature of the likely underlying condition?
   A. Myopia
   B. Lacrimal duct obstruction
   C. Macular hole
   D. Keratoconus

61) A 12-month-old girl is noted for having poor interaction behaviour. Ocular examination revealed reduced red reflex and bilateral cataracts. Which of the following is NOT a known risk factor?
   A. Toxoplasmosis
   B. Edwards syndrome
   C. Galactosaemia
   D. Homocystinuria

62) Which of the following is a Grade 3 of binocular vision?
   A. Stereopsis
   B. Simultaneous perception
   C. Fusion
   D. Suppression

63) An 8-year-old boy presents with swelling of his right eyelids and complains of ocular pain and double vision. Ocular examination revealed marked periocular erythema, conjunctival injection and reduced abduction in the right eye. Which of the following is the **MOST** suitable treatment?
   A. Metronidazole
   B. Co-amoxiclav
   C. Aciclovir
   D. Ciprofloxacin

64) A 7-year-old girl was brought in by her mother, who noticed a painless lump in the girl's right lower lid over the last few days. Which of the following structure is **MOST** likely involved?
   A. Gland of Moll
   B. Gland of Zeiss
   C. Meibomian gland
   D. Hair follicle

65) Which of the following is **NOT** a leading cause of childhood blindness in low-income countries?
   A. Congenital cataract
   B. Corneal scarring
   C. Glaucoma
   D. Retinopathy of prematurity

66) Which of the following is a side effect of acetazolamide?
   A. Metabolic alkalosis
   B. Metabolic acidosis
   C. Respiratory acidosis
   D. Respiratory alkalosis

67) A patient, who is normally fit and well, presents with raised intraocular pressure following a complicated cataract surgery with hyphaema and vitreous haemorrhage a month ago. Which of the following is the most likely underlying diagnosis?
   A. Phacolytic glaucoma
   B. Ghost cell "glaucoma"
   C. Angle recession glaucoma
   D. Schwartz-Matsuo syndrome

68) A patient cannot remember his glasses prescription. He tells you that he vaguely remembers his refraction as +6.50D or +6.00D, but he is not sure which is for his contact lenses and which is for his glasses. Which of these is **MORE** likely to be the power of his contact lenses and what is the relative image size when compared with his glasses?
   A. +6.00D; larger image
   B. +6.50D; smaller image
   C. +6.00D; smaller image
   D. +6.50D; larger image

69) Which of the following is the spherical equivalent of −2.00 / +1.00 × 90°?
   A. −1.00
   B. −1.50
   C. −2.50
   D. −3.00

70) Which part of the cornea does fluorescein stain?
   A. Epithelium
   B. Bowman layer
   C. Stroma
   D. Endothelium

71) Which of the following forms the outermost layer of the tear film?
   A. Aqueous
   B. Mucin
   C. Lipid
   D. Keratin

72) Which of the following is the **MOST COMMON** cause of infectious scleritis?
   A. Lyme disease
   B. *Pseudomonas aeruginosa*
   C. Herpes zoster
   D. Tuberculosis

73) A 7-year-old boy is brought in by his mother, who has noticed a blue tinge on the white of his eyes. Which of the following would **NOT** account for this presentation?
   A. Ehlers-Danlos syndrome
   B. Bardet-Biedl syndrome
   C. Osteogenesis imperfecta
   D. Alkaptonuria

74) A 31-year-old Japanese female has been referred by her GP to the eye clinic to investigate pigmentation of her right sclera. On examination her right sclera contains multiple diffuse grey areas of pigmentation. You also notice a deep bluish hyperpigmentation of the ipsilateral periocular skin. Which of the following is the **MOST LIKELY** underlying diagnosis?
   A. Ocular melanocytosis
   B. Dermal melanocytosis
   C. Primary acquired melanosis
   D. Naevus of Ota

75) Which of the following is the most common cause of eventual visual loss as a result of anterior scleritis?
   A. Perforation
   B. Glaucoma
   C. Peripheral ulcerative keratitis
   D. Hypotony

76) Which of the following embryonic tissues is the corneal epithelium derived from?
   A. Mesoderm
   B. Neuroectoderm
   C. Neural crest
   D. Surface ectoderm

77) The World Health Organisation (WHO) defines blindness as a visual acuity (Snellen score) of **less than**:
   A. 6/30
   B. 6/60
   C. 1/30
   D. 3/60

78) Ivermectin is indicated in the treatment of
   A. Syphilis
   B. Tuberculosis
   C. Cysticercosis
   D. Onchocerciasis

79) Which of the following results would be compatible with a diagnosis of keratoconjunctivitis sicca?
   A. Tear film break-up time of 15 seconds
   B. Schirmer 1 test of 8 mm
   C. Schirmer 2 test of 7 mm
   D. Tear film break-up time of 10 seconds

80) A 27-year-old contact lens wearer presents with a 5-day history of severe left eye pain and photophobia. On examination perineural infiltrates are seen. Which of the following is the **MOST LIKELY** diagnosis?
   A. Acanthamoeba keratitis
   B. Fungal keratitis
   C. HSV keratitis
   D. Bacterial keratitis

81) Innervation to the cornea is supplied by the:
   A. Long ciliary nerves
   B. Posterior ciliary nerves
   C. Short ciliary nerves
   D. Anterior ciliary nerves

82) Which of the following statements regarding allergic conjunctivitis is **TRUE**?
    A. Atopic keratoconjunctivitis (AKC) does not cause keratoconus
    B. Vernal keratoconjunctivitis (VKC) primarily affects middle-aged women
    C. AKC affects the inferior palpebral conjunctiva more than the superior
    D. It is a predominantly Type IV hypersensitivity reaction

83) In retinoblastoma, which of the following stages of the cell cycle is defective?
    A. S phase
    B. G1 phase
    C. M phase
    D. G2 phase

84) Which of the following is typically seen in a congenital cataract?
    A. Snowflake opacity
    B. Flower-shaped opacity
    C. Wedge-shaped/star-like opacity
    D. Lamellar opacity

85) Which of the following is **NOT** a feature of intraoperative floppy iris syndrome?
    A. Iris prolapse through incision sites
    B. Progressive pupillary constriction during surgery
    C. Intraoperative iris billowing
    D. Associated with the use of the timolol

86) What is the definition of prevalence?
    A. Average number of individuals who need to receive the treatment for one of them to get the positive outcome
    B. Proportion of new cases of a disease in a defined population during a specified time period
    C. Chance of a disease occurring in one group compared to another group
    D. Proportion of existing cases of a disease in a defined population at a given point in time

87) Which of the following is NOT associated with a displaced lens?
   A. Pseudoexfoliation
   B. Marfan syndrome
   C. Hypolysinaemia
   D. Homocystinuria

88) Which of the following is an age-related cataract in which the symptom of glare predominates?
   A. Nuclear sclerotic
   B. Punctate
   C. Cortical
   D. Coronary

89) Which of the following is FALSE regarding lens proteins?
   A. They constitute approximately 10% of the lens mass
   B. Beta crystallin is the main soluble protein
   C. Albuminoid is the main insoluble protein
   D. The concentration of insoluble proteins increases with age

90) Which of the following nerves carries autonomic fibres that are responsible for pupil dilation?
   A. Trochlear nerve
   B. Lacrimal nerve
   C. Frontal nerve
   D. Nasociliary nerve

91) Which of the following antibiotics inhibits protein synthesis?
   A. Penicillin
   B. Ciprofloxacin
   C. Doxycycline
   D. Trimethoprim

92) Which of the following is NOT a risk factor for retinal vein occlusion?
   A. Hypertension
   B. Glaucoma
   C. Cancer
   D. Atrial fibrillation

93) Which of the following would most likely result in superior displacement of the globe?
A. Maxillary carcinoma
B. Cavernous haemangioma
C. Encephalocoele
D. Optic nerve glioma

94) Which of the following regarding the annulus Zinn is **FALSE**?
A. The abducens nerve traverses it
B. The trochlear nerve traverses it
C. The medical rectus muscle originates from it
D. The superior rectus muscle originates from it

95) A 71-year-old male with diabetes undergoes uneventful cataract surgery. He has normal visual acuity for the first few days but then noticed a drop in visual acuity to 6/24 in the operated eye 3 weeks later. Preoperative examination was unremarkable apart from cataracts. What is the most likely diagnosis?
A. Age-related macular degeneration
B. Central serous chorioretinopathy
C. Macular hole
D. Cystoid macular oedema

96) Which of the following contributes to the mucin layer of the tear film?
A. Crypts of Henle
B. Glands of Krause
C. Glands of Wolfring
D. Meibomian glands

97) Which of the following is **NOT** an antagonist of right abduction?
A. Right medial rectus
B. Right superior rectus
C. Right superior oblique
D. Right inferior rectus

98) The nasolacrimal duct drains into the:
A. Inferior nasal meatus
B. Middle nasal meatus
C. Superior nasal meatus
D. Sphenoethmoidal recess

99) Which of the following structures exits the skull at the foramen ovale?
   A. Maxillary nerve
   B. Mandibular nerve
   C. Middle meningeal artery
   D. Greater petrosal nerve

100) Which of the following segments of the optic nerve has the longest course?
   A. Intraocular
   B. Intracanalicular
   C. Intraorbital
   D. Intracranial

Mock Exam Paper Answers

1) A
The investigation findings described are suggestive of primary open-angle glaucoma (POAG), whereby optic disc cupping and pallor are noted. Bayonetting of vessels refers to the breaks seen in vessels as they disappear into the deep cup and reappear at the base. First-line treatment for POAG is a class of drug known as prostaglandins such as latanoprost and bimatoprost. Beta-blockers (e.g., timolol) are usually a second-line therapy for POAG. However, in this case, it is contraindicated as the patient is known to suffer from asthma.

2) B
The lens dioptre (D) refers to the curvature of the lens. As the dioptre increases, the lens becomes thicker and the curvature greater. As the curvature increases, the light rays are redirected to fill a greater portion of the viewer's retina, which makes the object look bigger, and thus the magnification.

There are a few formulae to convert the dioptre of a lens into its magnification but a quick way of finding the approximate magnification is:

- Magnification = Dioptre ÷ 4 + 1

In this case, for a 16D lens of a magnifier, its magnification = 16/4 + 1 = 5x. Hence objects viewed under a 16D lens will appear 5x larger than normal.

3) A
The first step in the management of a childhood squint, particularly an esotropia (which is often due to an uncorrected hypermetropic refractive error), is to perform a cycloplegic refraction and correct any refractive error with appropriate glasses. Often, once the child has adapted to their glasses, the squint subsides.

4) B
Traumatic entrapment of an extraocular muscle results in mechanical restriction, which does not improve with the cover-uncover test. In the case of a left lateral rectus muscle entrapment, this will result in the inability to adduct the left eye. Consecutive exotropia refers to a divergent strabismus that commonly develops following surgical correction of an esotropia. It may also develop spontaneously in an amblyopic eye. The most common scenario is an adult who had childhood surgery for an infantile esotropia, whose eyes were straight for many years, but then develops a divergent strabismus in later life.

Duane retraction syndrome is a congenital eye movement anomaly characterised by variable horizontal duction deficits, with narrowing of the palpebral fissure and globe retraction on attempted adduction, occasionally accompanied by an upshoot or downshoot of the globe.

A lesion in the medial longitudinal fasciculus is responsible for the clinical presentation of internuclear ophthalmoplegia (INO) and is most commonly associated with demyelinating causes such as multiple sclerosis. The eyes are straight in a primary gaze and there is a defective adduction of the eye on the side of the lesion and an ataxic nystagmus of the contralateral eye on abduction. Therefore, in the case of a right INO, there will be reduced adduction of the right eye on a left gaze (as opposed to the description in this case).

5) A
Prostaglandin analogues, such as latanoprost, are typically avoided in patients with concurrent inflammatory conditions, such as in the case of acute angle-closure glaucoma, due to the potential to exacerbate inflammation. It is also believed that the onset of pressure reduction action of prostaglandin analogues is generally unacceptably slow to be of any value in an acute situation.

6) D
In order to achieve emmetropia, the required spectacle prescription will be acting in the opposite magnitude and axis to the patient's own optical refractive error.

In this case, a spectacle correction of −1.50 / +3.00 × 90° will neutralise the patient's astigmatism of +1.50 / −3.00 × 180°.

7) A
A pachymeter (the prefix pachy is derived from the ancient Greek work pachys, which means thick) is a device used to measure corneal

thickness. This can be done using either optical or ultrasonic pachymetry.

8) D

Prostaglandin analogues can be favourable to beta-blockers as they are more potent and have fewer systemic side effects. However, the most commonly observed side effects include:

- Conjunctival hyperaemia
- Increase in iris pigmentation (D)
- Increase in eyelash length

A reduction in vision in patients with cataracts (A) can be seen with the use of pilocarpine.

9) D

The above scenario describes the Parks 3-step test (also known as Parks-Bielschowsky 3-step test), which is a diagnostic test used to isolate the paretic muscle in acquired vertical diplopia. It uses the cover-uncover test, with or without the Maddox rod to measure the amount of deviation in different head positions. It is unreliable when there are multiple paretic muscles or in restrictive strabismus.

The three steps as applied to the scenario above is:

- Step 1: Which eye is hyperdeviated in primary gaze?

    If the left eye is the hyperdeviated eye, we know that the failing muscle is either responsible for depressing the left eye or elevating the right eye. Our suspects are therefore:

    Left eye: Left superior oblique (LSO) or left inferior rectus (LIR)
    Right eye: Right superior rectus (RSR) or right inferior oblique (RIO)

- Step 2: Is the vertical deviation greater in the right or left gaze?

    When we look in the right gaze the muscles most responsible for the eyes' vertical position are the right rectus muscles and the left oblique muscles. As the hypertropia is worse in the right gaze, we know that our suspects are:

    Left eye: LSO or left inferior oblique (LIO)
    Right eye: RSR or right inferior rectus (RIR)

- Step 3: Is the vertical deviation greater with a right head tilt or left head tilt?

When the head is tilted to the left, the right eye needs to turn outward (excyclotorsion) and the left eye needs to turn inward (incyclotorsion). As the deviation is worse in the left head tilt, the muscles responsible for these movements (and are therefore suspects) are:

Left eye: LSO or LSR
Right eye: RIO or RIR

Result: Based on the 3-step test, the only extraocular muscle NOT eliminated in each step is the LSO, which is therefore the paretic muscle.

10) A

Optic disc drusen are intra- and extracellular deposits (often calcified) that accumulate within the optic nerve head. They occur in 0.4% of children and often pose a diagnostic dilemma as they may simulate papilloedema. Patients are usually asymptomatic, with optic disc drusen being detected incidentally. Diagnosis is usually based on clinical examination with the aid of ancillary testing such as B-scan ultrasonography, which will classically show hyperechoic signal(s) at the optic nerve head.

11) D

Capillary haemangioma (strawberry naevus) is one of the most common benign tumours in children. It is more common in girls and usually presents as a unilateral, raised bright red lesion on the upper lid within 6 months of life. Ptosis is frequent and the lesion may expand on crying. The majority of capillary haemangiomas around the eye do not require intervention and can be monitored.

Pyogenic granuloma is a rapidly growing vascularised proliferation of granulation tissue that is usually preceded by surgery, trauma or infection. Clinically, there is a painful, rapidly growing, vascular granulating lesion that may bleed following relatively trivial trauma.

Cavernous haemangioma is the most common orbital tumour in adults, with a female preponderance of 70%. It occurs in middle-aged adults and usually presents as slowly progressive unilateral proptosis.

Cutaneous neurofibromas are benign nerve tumours, usually nodular or pedunculated, that can be found anywhere on the skin. Isolated neurofibromas are common in normal individuals, but if multiple lesions are present, neurofibromatosis should be excluded.

Plexiform neurofibromas typically present in childhood as a manifestation of neurofibromatosis type 1 with a characteristic S-shaped deformity of the upper eyelid.

12) B

When administered exogenously, corticosteroids increase the risk of glaucoma by increasing intraocular pressure. They also increase the risk of developing posterior subcapsular cataracts. Amiodarone (A) is associated with vortex keratopathy (also known as cornea verticillata), whereby corneal deposits are seen at the level of the basal epithelium. It can also cause optic neuropathy, which affects 1–2% of patients on long-term amiodarone treatment. Digoxin (B) is associated with abnormal colour vision but is not known to cause vortex keratopathy. Vigabatrin (an antiepileptic) (D) is associated with visual field defects.

13) C

The Watzke-Allen test is used as a diagnostic clinical test for the detection of macular holes. The Ishihara test is the most widely used colour vision test due to its wide availability and ease of usage. It is designed to screen for congenital protan and deutan defects. It consists of a test plate followed by 16 plates, which contain a central number or shape contained within a matrix of coloured dots. The Farnsworth-Munsell 100-hue test is more sensitive but takes longer to perform. Despite the name, it consists of 85 caps of different hues in four racks. The patient is asked to rearrange randomised caps in order of colour progression, and the findings are recorded on a circular chart.

The Hardy-Rand-Rittler test is similar to the Ishihara test but can detect all three congenital colour defects (protan, deutan and tritan).

14) B

Retinoblastoma is the most common primary intraocular malignancy of childhood. The most common presentation is usually with leukocoria (white pupillary reflex), followed by strabismus. The mean age of diagnosis is 1 year for bilateral retinoblastoma and 2 years for unilateral retinoblastoma. A large majority of heritable retinoblastoma (about 40% of cases) develop bilateral and multifocal tumours.

Persistent fetal vasculature (also known as persistent hyperplastic primary vitreous) is a congenital unilateral developmental anomaly characterised by the persistence of embryologic mesenchymal tissue remnants in the vitreous cavity.

Coats disease is an idiopathic condition that is characterised by pathologic telangiectatic retinal vessels that leak and lead to an accumulation of subretinal fluid and exudate, which may present as leukocoria. It is almost always unilateral and tends to present later than retinoblastoma.

Retinopathy of prematurity results from the failure of development of the normal retina in premature neonates exposed to high levels of oxygen during the postnatal period. There is usually a clear history of prematurity and low birth weight.

15) A
Sturge-Weber syndrome (encephalotrigeminal angiomatosis) is a congenital, sporadic phacomatosis that affects the meninges and facial skin. Involvement is usually unilateral and due to the failure of embryonic blood vessels to regress during development. This results in the formation of angiomas on the face, meninges and ipsilateral eye. The angiomas on the face are referred to as port-wine stains and are well demarcated and non-blanching. They often present in the ophthalmic and maxillary divisions of the trigeminal nerve. Leptomeningeal haemangioma involving the central nervous system may cause focal or generalised seizures, hemiparesis or hemianopia.

16) B
Optic nerve hypoplasia arises from the underdevelopment of the optic nerve. Young maternal age, maternal diabetes and alcohol are associated with an increased risk of optic nerve hypoplasia. Visual acuity can range from normal to perception of light; severe bilateral cases present with blindness in early infancy with roving eye movements or nystagmus.

Leber hereditary optic neuropathy is a rare ganglion cell degeneration, which is caused by maternally inherited mitochondrial DNA mutations. This condition typically affects males between the ages of 15 and 35 years.

Central serous chorioretinopathy is a fluid detachment of the macula where there is an accumulation of subretinal fluid. It typically occurs in males between the ages of 20 to 50 years and presents with acute or subacute central vision loss or distortion.

Nutritional optic neuropathy (tobacco-alcohol amblyopia) is an acquired optic neuropathy and typically affects individuals with high alcohol and tobacco consumption.

17) B
The image formed by a prism is always erect, virtual and deviated towards the apex.

18) C
The definitive investigation in infective endophthalmitis is microscopy, culture and sensitivity (MC&S) tests performed on vitreous specimens. A polymerase chain reaction (PCR) can also be performed on the sample to detect genetic material. An anterior chamber tap (A) can also be used to investigate infective endophthalmitis but is of lower yield. Corneal scrapes (D) are used to investigate corneal ulcers.

19) D
Central retinal vein occlusion (D) is most likely to present with a sudden (rather than gradual) painless loss of vision. The fundal appearance is typically that of scattered flame-shaped haemorrhages and cotton wool spots on the retina.

20) A
A cylindrical (toric) lens is used in the correction of regular astigmatism. It has one plane surface and one cylindrical (and hence only one meridian of curvature). The plane surface represents the axis, which does not have any power. The cylindrical (curved) surface is 90 degrees to the plane surface (axis) and has maximum refractive power that forms a focal line parallel to its axis.

21) C
A spectacle prescription may be written in plus or minus cylinder notation (i.e., the second number in the prescription can either be plus or minus). These are the two equivalent ways in which any single refractive error can be corrected.

To obtain the equivalent notation, one form has to be transposed to the other (i.e., transposing plus to minus cylinder notation or vice versa). This involves three steps:

1. Add the spherical and cylindrical power to give the new sphere
2. Change the sign of the cylinder power
3. Add 90 degrees to the existing axis, as the new axis will be perpendicular to the old axis. (NB. If the axis is more than 180

degrees, minus 180 degrees from the total degrees to get the new axis.)

Therefore, transposing −2.00 / +1.00 x 120°:

1. New sphere = (−2.00) + (+1.00) = −1.00
2. New cylinder = −1.00
3. New axis
    - 120° + 90° = 210° (add 90 degrees to the existing axis)
    - 210° − 180° = 30° (as the new axis is more than 180 degrees, 180 degrees is deducted from it to give the new axis)

This gives a transposition equivalent of −1.00 / −1.00 x 30°.

22) C

Age-related macular degeneration (C) presents with painless vision loss and metamorphopsia and is not associated with painful or red eyes. Important causes of a red eye include conjunctivitis, acute angle-closure glaucoma, acute anterior uveitis, trauma, keratitis, scleritis and episcleritis.

23) C

The most likely diagnosis in this case is multiple sclerosis (MS). Optic neuritis is the presenting feature in about a third of patients with MS. In addition to changes in the optic nerve appearance, an MRI would almost always reveal characteristic lesions in the white matter of the brain. Disease-modifying therapies such as interferon beta, natalizumab, glatiramer acetate and fingolimod are used in the long-term management of MS. They are steroid-sparing and can prevent relapses and reduce neurological disability.

Although there is evidence to suggest small improvements from treatment with methotrexate in patients with MS, larger studies are still ongoing to investigate whether the benefits of this drug outweigh its potentially serious side effects.

24) D

A focimeter (also known as a lensmeter) is used to measure the power and axes (if the cylindrical component is present) of a lens. It can also be used to locate the optical centre of a lens and quantify the power of any incorporated prism.

25) B

In myopia, the second principal focus lies in front of the retina. Myopia may be classified into axial myopia (in which the eye is abnormally long such as in the presence of a posterior staphyloma) or refractive/index myopia (in which the refractive power of the eye is increased such as in nucleosclerosis or keratoconus).

Central serous chorioretinopathy may induce hypermetropia (rather than myopia) due to the elevation of the fovea from subretinal fluid. Myopia can be addressed by clear lens extraction, in which the original crystalline lens is removed and replaced with an intraocular lens.

26) C

The image formed by the indirect ophthalmoscope is real and inverted (both horizontally and vertically). It is relatively unaffected by the refractive state of the patient's eye compared to direct ophthalmoscopy.

27) B

Propionibacterium acnes is the most common cause of delayed-onset postoperative endophthalmitis. This low virulence bacterium can become sequestered within macrophages where it is protected from eradication but continues to express the bacterial antigen. There is usually a delayed onset postoperatively, which ranges from 4 weeks to years (the mean is 9 months).

Staphylococcus epidermidis is the most common cause of acute postoperative endophthalmitis.

28) C

Achromatopsia (congenital monochromatism) is a group of congenital disorders in which there is reduced visual acuity and an inability to perceive colours. There are two main subtypes: (1) complete achromatopsia (rod monochromatism) and (2) incomplete achromatopsia (blue cone monochromatism). There is full impairment of the cone function in the former, whereas there is partial impairment of the cone function (only blue cones are functioning and hence the term blue cone monochromatism) in the latter. Rod cell function is retained in achromatopsia.

29) B

The word "laser" is an acronym for "light amplification by stimulated emission of radiation". It has particular use in ophthalmology due to the transparent nature of the cornea, which allows light such as laser to reach almost all the tissues of the eye.

30) C
CT is generally the preferred imaging modality as it is better than X-ray at detecting and pinpointing the location of radiopaque foreign bodies. Non-radiopaque foreign bodies may be determined by an experienced ultrasonographer but is contraindicated if there is any evidence of a ruptured globe from a penetrating injury. An MRI is contraindicated as the magnetic force may cause severe ocular damage should the foreign body be metallic in nature.

31) A
Atropine is a muscarinic antagonist. The onset of mydriasis precedes that of cycloplegia and tends to last longer. It has a longer duration of action (up to 2 weeks) compared to tropicamide (4–8 hours) and cyclopentolate (24 hours).

32) C
Hypocalcaemia (rather than hypercalcaemia) is associated with cataract formation. The other options are known metabolic causes of cataract.

33) B
The main proteins of the human lens are alpha, beta and gamma crystallins. The anterior sutures are in the shape of an upright Y, whereas the posterior sutures are an inverted Y. The anterior lens capsule thickens with age, whereas the posterior lens capsule changes minimally throughout life.

34) A
The Nd:YAG (neodymium-doped yttrium aluminium garnet) laser is accepted as the standard treatment in laser capsulotomy for posterior capsular opacification, which can occur after cataract surgery.

35) C
Rod cells are almost entirely responsible for night vision. In cone-rod dystrophy, visual acuity and colour vision loss precede night blindness and peripheral vision loss due to the loss of cone cells first. The other options (Best disease, Stargardt disease and cone dystrophy) are different forms of macular dystrophy, which involve progressive generalised cone dysfunction.

36) B

Optical radiation consists of ultraviolet, visible radiation and infrared. It lies between X-rays and microwaves on the electromagnetic spectrum. Radio waves and gamma rays have the longest and shortest wavelength, respectively, on the electromagnetic spectrum.

37) D

Refraction is defined as the change in direction of light when it passes from one transparent medium into another with different optical density. On entering an optically denser medium from a less dense medium (i.e., from air into glass), light is deviated towards the normal. The angle of refraction (r) in such a situation will therefore be less than that of the angle of incidence (i) (see figure below).

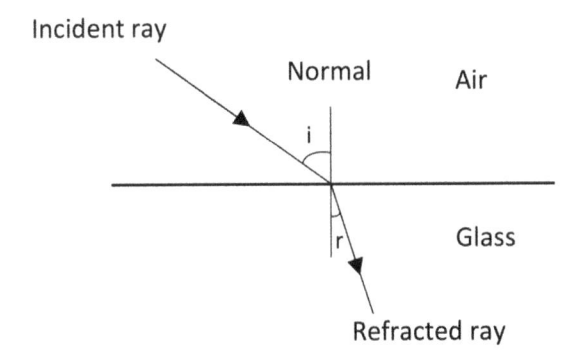

Refraction of light entering an optically denser medium (glass) from air

38) D

Each colour has a specific frequency and wavelength. The relationship between the frequency and wavelength for electromagnetic waves is defined by the formula, $c = \lambda f$, where c is the speed of light, λ the wavelength in metres, and f equals the frequency in cycles per second.

39) A

Laser light is nearly monochromatic and consists of essentially one wavelength, having its origin in stimulated emission from one set of atomic energy level.

40) B

Monovision (or blended vision) is a type of vision where the vision in the dominant eye is corrected for distance vision (i.e., emmetropic), while the other eye is intentionally left slightly myopic to allow viewing of close objects. This allows both eyes to work together and to see clearly at any distance. It is mainly reserved for patients who have developed presbyopia. However, due to the use of only one eye for a particular distance, it may reduce binocular visual acuity and stereopsis.

41) A
The slit lamp can be used to examine the fundus. This is achieved by using a condensing lens, which offers a high resolution and stereoscopic view.

42) C
Optical coherence tomography angiography (OCT-A), rather than standard OCT, is a non-invasive technique for the imaging of retinal and choroidal circulation.

43) B
In oblique astigmatism, the axis of the correcting cylinder is either near 90 degrees or 180 degrees (i.e., with- or against-the-rule astigmatism, respectively).

44) C
The lens and the cornea are the two main refractive elements of the human eye. The average optic power of the human eye is 60D, of which the cornea accounts for approximately two thirds (43D) and the lens one third (17D). The anterior lens surface is less curved (and hence a longer radius of curvature) than the posterior lens surface. The lens has different refractive indexes within its substance, while the nucleus tends to have a higher refractive index than the cortex.

45) D
Convex (plus-powered) and concave (minus-powered) spectacle lenses magnify and minify images in hypermetropia and myopia, respectively. As contact lenses tend to return the images to near-normal size, the images are minified in hypermetropia and magnified in myopia when transitioning from spectacle lenses.

46) A
The crab louse *Phthirus pubis* is an insect that is usually found in a person's pubic hair. In children, *Phthirus pubis* may be found in their eyelashes and can be a sign of sexual abuse.

Pediculosis capitis is a head louse. *Demodex folliculorum* is a common hair follicle and sebaceous gland dwelling mite — reaction to this may play a causative role for blepharitis in some patients. *Borrelia burgdorferi* is a bacterium responsible for Lyme disease.

47) B
The main bacterial pathogens (in descending order of frequency) in children are *Haemophilus influenzae, Streptococcus pneumoniae, Staphylococcus aureus* and *Moraxella catarrhalis.*

48) C
Retinitis pigmentosa refers to a clinically and genetically diverse group of inherited diffuse retinal degenerative diseases initially affecting the rod photoreceptors, with later degeneration of cones (rod-cone dystrophy). It may occur as a sporadic disorder, or be inherited in an autosomal dominant, autosomal recessive or X-linked recessive (XLR) pattern. XLR is the least common but most severe form and may result in complete blindness by the 3rd or 4th decade of life.

49) D
Cytomegalovirus (CMV) is the most common congenital infection in infants. At least 90% of adults in developed countries show past exposure to CMV, which is usually acquired during the first 5 years of life. It is usually subclinical but ocular features may include cataract, microphthalmos, chorioretinitis, optic disc hypoplasia and optic atrophy.

50) A
Juvenile idiopathic arthritis is by far the most common systemic disease associated with childhood anterior uveitis. Both eyes are affected in 70% of patients.

51) B
Nasolacrimal duct obstruction (NLDO) is a common ocular condition in infants with spontaneous resolution in over 90% within the first year. Gentle lacrimal sac massage with a hot compress is the usual first-line treatment for NLDO, failing which punctal dilation and probing should be considered.

52) A
The optic nerve enters the orbit through the optic canal, which is adjacent to the superior orbital fissure.

53) D
The Lang test is used to measure stereopsis.

The Hirschberg test provides a rough objective estimate of the angle of a manifest strabismus and is particularly useful in young or uncooperative patients.

The Krimsky test is a modified version of the Hirschberg test in which prisms are employed to provide a more accurate approximate of the angle of a manifest strabismus.

The prism cover test measures the angle of deviation on near or distance fixation. It combines the alternate cover test with prisms.

54) B
Parinaud syndrome (also known as dorsal midbrain syndrome) is characterised by the classic triad of: (1) upward gaze palsy, (2) pupillary light-near dissociation and (3) convergence-retraction nystagmus. Common causes in children include pinealoma and aqueductal stenosis. In adults, demyelination, infarction and tumours are more common causes. It is not known to be associated with chronic progressive external ophthalmoplegia.

55) A
The orbital floor is the most common location for orbital blowout fractures. Its close proximity to the inferior rectus muscle means that there is a risk of entrapment of this muscle with subsequent restriction of upward gaze.

56) C
The medial rectus muscle inserts closest to the limbus (5.5 mm from the limbus) compared to the other recti muscles (inferior rectus — 6.5 mm; lateral rectus — 6.9 mm; and superior rectus — 7.7 mm). It is also the largest of the extraocular muscles, with its size probably resulting from the frequency of its use in convergence.

57) B
Laser in situ keratomileusis (LASIK) involves creating a corneal flap using a microkeratome or a femtosecond laser. The underlying stromal bed is then ablated and reshaped using an excimer laser with the flap subsequently replaced. LASIK patients tend to spend less time recovering as it is only the edges of the flap that need to heal. However,

flap-related complications (e.g., epithelial ingrowth, diffuse lamellar keratitis) may be an issue.

58) D
Oral lutein is a supplement that has been shown to reduce the risk of age-related macular degeneration.

59) C
The forehead is typically spared in supranuclear brainstem lesions of the facial nerve. This is because the upper motor neurones for the upper face (e.g., upper portions of the orbicularis oculi and frontalis muscles of the forehead) project to the facial nuclei bilaterally.

Lesions of CN VII in the posterior fossa (cerebellopontine angle) such as acoustic neuroma and meningioma result in ipsilateral lower motor neurone facial nerve paralysis (including loss of taste over the ipsilateral anterior two thirds of the tongue) without hyperacusis. Due to the close proximity to CN VIII, there may also be ipsilateral tinnitus, deafness and vertigo.

Involvement of the geniculate ganglion results in ipsilateral facial motor paralysis, loss of taste over the anterior two thirds of the tongue and hyperacusis (due to stapedius muscle paralysis).

Lesions in the facial canal distal to the departure of the chorda tympani (e.g., lesions at the stylomastoid foramen) cause facial motor paralysis without associated hyperacusis or loss of taste.

60) C
Down syndrome (trisomy 21) is usually characterised by specific facial features (i.e., upslanting palpebral fissures, large epicanthic folds), short stature, intellectual disability and cardiac anomalies. Individuals with Down syndrome are at increased risk of a wide range of ocular disorders, which include refractive errors, strabismus, nystagmus, cataracts, lacrimal duct obstruction, keratoconus and blepharitis. A macular hole is not a known ocular feature.

61) D
Congenital cataracts are responsible for up to 20% of child blindness worldwide and the majority of bilateral congenital cataracts are idiopathic. It is however important to exclude causes such as metabolic disorders (e.g., galactosaemia), intrauterine infections (**TORCH**; **TO**xoplasmosis, **R**ubella, **C**ytomegalovirus, **H**erpes simplex) and systemic associations

(e.g., Down and Edwards syndrome). Homocystinuria is not associated with congenital cataract(s) but rather ectopia lentis.

62) A

There are 3 grades of binocular vision in Worth's classification, which can be graded on a synoptophore:

Grade 1: Simultaneous Perception	This is the most elementary binocularity. It occurs when the visual cortex perceives separate stimuli to the two eyes at the same time
Grade 2: Fusion	Both eyes are able to produce a composite picture (sensory fusion) from two similar images
Grade 3: Stereopsis	This is the highest type of binocularity where there is an ability to obtain an impression of depth by the superimposition of two images

63) B

The above scenario describes orbital cellulitis, which is an ophthalmic emergency. Clinical presentation is typically with a painful, red eye associated with periocular swelling, proptosis and ophthalmoplegia. It most commonly occurs when bacterial infection (*Haemophilus influenzae, Streptococcus, Staphylococcus aureus*) spreads from the adjacent paranasal sinuses, most often from the ethmoid sinus through the thin lamina papyracea of the medial orbital wall. It may cause blindness and progress to life-threatening sequelae such as brain abscess, meningitis and cavernous sinus thrombosis. Successful management is, therefore, dependent upon immediate treatment. This involves prompt admission with the initiation of systemic antibiotics (such as co-amoxiclav) and a multi-disciplinary approach with paediatricians and ENT surgeons.

64) C

This lump is most likely to represent a chalazion, which results from blocked meibomian glands. It is typically painless and not red.

A stye (also known as an external hordeolum), on the other hand, is a red, painful lump that usually results from an infected hair follicle.

A cyst of Zeiss is a small benign, non-translucent cyst arising from a gland of Zeiss. It is filled with sebaceous material.

A cyst of Moll (also known as apocrine hidrocystoma) is a small, benign, translucent cyst arising from obstruction of the apocrine secretory duct of the gland of Moll.

65) D

According to the WHO, corneal scarring (secondary to measles, vitamin A deficiency, use of harmful traditional eye remedies and ophthalmia neonatorum) and congenital cataract (secondary to rubella infection) are the major causes of childhood blindness in low-income countries.

In middle-income countries, retinopathy of prematurity is an important cause of childhood blindness, whereas optic nerve and higher visual pathways pathology predominate as the cause of blindness in high-income countries.

Other significant causes in all countries include congenital abnormalities such as glaucoma and hereditary retinal dystrophies.

66) B

Carbonic anhydrase inhibitors (both topical and systemic) such as acetazolamide are frequently used in the management of raised intraocular pressure. One of its main side effects is metabolic acidosis due to the inhibitory effect on the reabsorption of bicarbonate (HCO^{-3}) ions from renal tubules.

67) B

Ghost cell "glaucoma" refers to raised intraocular pressure (IOP) where there is trabecular obstruction by degenerate red blood cells. It usually occurs a few weeks after a vitreous haemorrhage.

Angle recession glaucoma is classically a sequela of previous blunt trauma, whereas phacolytic glaucoma is associated with a hypermature cataract.

Schwartz-Matsuo syndrome refers to raised IOP in patients with rhegmatogenous retinal detachment. The aetiology is believed to be displaced photoreceptor outer segments compromising trabecular outflow.

68) B

Lens effectivity is the change in the vergence of light that occurs at different points along its path. This is related to vertex distance, which is the distance between the back surface of a corrective lens (i.e., spectacles or contact lenses) and the front of the cornea. For spectacles, placing a minus lens closer to the eyes increases the effective power of the lens (more −). The converse is true for plus lens; moving it away from the eyes increases the effective power of the lens (more +).

The closer to the eye the lens is mounted, the shorter its focal length in the case of hypermetropia, and the longer its focal length in the case of myopia. Because of this, plus power has to be added in both cases. Therefore, hypermetropes need more plus (and vice versa — myopes need less minus) when going from spectacles to contact lens. A useful mnemonic to remember this rule is **CAP — Close Add Plus**.

In a hypermetropic patient, spectacle lenses (which will be convex in nature) have a magnifying effect on the patient's vision. The higher the degree of hypermetropia, the more the magnification effect of the corrective lenses. As contact lenses sit close to the eyes, the magnifying effect is lessened, and thus the perceived image will be smaller relative to that of spectacles. The converse is true for minus (concave) lenses; the perceived image with contact lens will be larger relative to that of spectacles.

69) B

The spherical equivalent is a quick and useful method to decide if an eye is overall myopic or hypermetropic. It combines the effect of the sphere and cylinder using the formula:

- Spherical equivalent: sphere + (cylinder ÷ 2)

The spherical equivalent can be obtained from the refractive prescription in either the plus or the minus cylinder format.

Taking the given prescription as an example, the spherical equivalent would be −2.00 + (+1.00 ÷ 2) = −1.50. This eye would be considered to be overall myopic.

70) C

To visualise corneal epithelial defects, fluorescein dye is instilled and visualised using a cobalt-blue filter, which causes the dye to fluoresce in a bright green colour. Fluorescein does not stain intact corneal epithelium but stains corneal stroma, thus demarcating the area of epithelial loss.

71) C

The tear film is composed of three layers:

- An outer lipid layer containing secretions from the meibomian glands

- A middle aqueous layer containing proteins, electrolytes and water secreted from the lacrimal glands
- An inner mucin layer derived from conjunctival goblet cells

72) C
All of the options are causes of infectious scleritis. However, herpes zoster is the most common infective cause. Other causes include leprosy, syphilis and *Nocardia*.

73) B
Major associations for blue scleral discolouration include osteogenesis imperfecta (types I and IIA) and Ehlers-Danlos syndrome. Alkaptonuria (an autosomal recessive disorder) can also cause a bluish-grey (or black) scleral pigmentation. Other more rare associations include Marshall-Smith syndrome and Russell-Silver syndrome.

74) D
Naevus of Ota (oculodermal melanocytosis) is the most common type of congenital ocular melanocytosis and involves both the eye and skin. It occurs commonly in Asians but rarely in white individuals. The involvement of the facial skin is often in the distribution of the first and second trigeminal divisions.

Dermal melanocytosis involves only the skin, whereas ocular melanocytosis involves only the eye.

Primary acquired melanosis (PAM) of the conjunctiva can be divided into (1) PAM without cellular atypia (benign intraepithelial proliferation of epithelial melanocytes) and (2) PAM with severe cellular atypia (melanoma *in situ* that has a high risk of progression to invasive melanoma). It usually presents in a middle-aged, white individual.

75) B
Complications of anterior scleritis include the following:

- Acute infiltrative stromal keratitis
- Sclerosing keratitis
- Peripheral ulcerative keratitis
- Uveitis
- Glaucoma
- Hypotony
- Perforation of the sclera

Of these, glaucoma is the most common cause of eventual loss of vision.

76) D

The embryological origin of the different structures of the eye can be remembered using the table below:

Endoderm	Mesoderm	Neural Crest	Ectoderm	
			Neural	Surface
Not in Eye	Extraocular muscles, Trabecular meshwork and Schlemm canal, Ciliary body, Vitreous, Choroid		• Optic nerve (ON) • Retina (neurosensory retina and retinal pigment epithelium) • Ciliary body and iris epithelium • Iris muscles	• Eyelids and eyelashes • Tear system: lacrimal gland, nasolacrimal system, meibomian gland • Conjunctiva • Corneal epithelium • Lens
	• Iris • ON sheath • Orbicularis oculi • Scleral and choroidal blood vessels	• Stroma (cornea and iris) • Sclera • Corneal endothelium and Descemet membrane • Bony orbit		

77) D

The WHO defines "low vision" as a visual acuity of less than 6/18 but equal or better than 3/60. Visual acuity of less than 3/60 is defined as blindness.

78) D

Onchocerciasis is caused by the parasitic helminth *Onchocerca volvulus* and is the second most common cause of infectious blindness in the world (the first being trachoma, which is caused by *Chlamydia trachomatis*). Ivermectin is the mainstay of treatment for onchocerciasis.

79) B

Keratoconjunctivitis sicca refers to dry eye disease of any severity and can either be attributed to aqueous tear deficiency (e.g., Sjögren syndrome) or evaporative tear dysfunction (e.g., meibomian gland dysfunction, low blink rate, contact lens wear).

Although no clinical tests allow the definitive diagnosis of dry eye, those that attempt to confirm and quantify include the following:

Tear Film Break-up Time	• Instillation of fluorescein into fornix • Time from last blink to first dry patch • <10 s = abnormal
Schirmer Test	• Filter paper behind the lower lid margin with eyes shut for 5 minutes • Schirmer 1[1]: <10 mm = abnormal • Schirmer 2[2]: <6mm = abnormal [1]Without topical anaesthesia: both basic and reflex secretion are measured [2]With topical anaesthesia: only basic secretion is measured

80) A

Acanthamoeba spp. are ubiquitous protozoa that can cause severe keratitis in contact lens wearer, especially if tap water is used for rinsing. Presentation is with blurred vision and severe pain that is usually disproportionate to the clinical signs. Perineural infiltrates (radial keratoneuritis) are pathognomonic.

81) A

Innervation to the cornea is via the long ciliary nerves (from the nasociliary branch of V_1). Nerves pass radially forward within the corneal stroma, before branching anteriorly to finish as free nerve endings.

82) C

VKC and AKC are two subtypes of allergic conjunctivitis. The table below outlines the key differences between the two. Conjunctival involvement in AKC is worse in the inferior palpebral area (C), whereas it is worse superiorly in VKC. Both AKC and VKC can cause keratoconus as a result of chronic eye rubbing. Allergic conjunctivitis is predominantly a Type I hypersensitivity reaction.

Vernal Keratoconjunctivitis (VKC)	• Primarily affects boys from 5 years old, resolves by adolescence in the majority of cases • Common in warm dry climates • Occurs on a seasonal basis: spring and summer • Sx: intense itching, lacrimation, photophobia • Conjunctival scrapings: abundant eosinophils • Palpebral, limbal and mixed subtypes • Disease is worse in superior palpebral conjunctiva
Atopic Keratoconjunctivitis (AKC)	• Male = Female • Develops in adulthood (30–50 years) • History of atopy • Perennial, worse in winter • Conjunctival scrapings: less eosinophils than VKC • Disease is worse in inferior palpebral conjunctiva

83) B

Mutations of the tumour suppressor gene *RB1* are responsible for most cases of retinoblastoma. One of the many roles of *the RB1* gene is to restrict a cell's ability to replicate DNA by preventing its progression from the G1 (Gap 1) to S (synthesis) phase of the cell division cycle.

84) D

Lamellar opacities occur either in the anterior or posterior lamella of the lens and usually extend radially. They can be sporadic or inherited in an autosomal dominant pattern. There may also be an association with intrauterine infections and metabolic disorders.

Snowflake cortical opacities are seen in a classic diabetic cataract. Flower-shaped opacity is usually a result of blunt trauma. Wedge-shaped/star-like opacity is typically seen in myotonic dystrophy.

85) D
Systemic alpha-blockers (rather than beta-blockers) such as tamsulosin are associated with intraoperative floppy iris syndrome (IFIS). Interestingly, suspending these medications preoperatively does not reduce the risk of IFIS. The other options form the triad that defines IFIS.

86) D
(A) refers to the number needed to treat, (B) refers to incidence, and (C) refers to the odds ratio.

87) C
Hyperlysinaemia (rather than hypolysinaemia) is associated with ectopia lentis.

88) C
A cortical cataract is an age-related cataract. As with a posterior subcapsular cataract, glare is a common symptom. Nuclear sclerotic cataract, on the other hand, is often associated with a myopic shift due to an increase in the refractive index of the nucleus.

Punctate (also known as blue dot) and coronary cataracts are types of congenital cataracts that are usually visually insignificant.

89) A
Albuminoid is the main insoluble protein of the lens. They increase in concentration with age and can result in light scattering and contribute to cataract formation. As for the soluble proteins of the lens, beta crystallin is the most common (51%), followed by alpha (31%) and then gamma (2%). All in all, proteins constitute about a third of the lens mass.

90) D
The nasociliary branch of the ophthalmic division of the trigeminal nerve (V_1) carries sympathetic fibres that innervate the dilator pupillae muscle.

91) C
Doxycycline belongs to the class of antibiotics called tetracyclines. They bind to the 30S ribosomal unit of bacteria, disrupt amino acyl tRNA binding and inhibit protein synthesis.

92) D

Retinal vein occlusion is most commonly associated with prothrombotic risk factors (as opposed to retinal artery occlusion, which is associated with embolic risk factors such as atrial fibrillation). Risk factors include:

- Older age
- Hypertension
- Diabetes
- Glaucoma
- Hypermetropia
- Hypercoagulable states (either acquired such as cancer or hereditary such as Factor V Leiden)

93) A

Maxillary carcinoma is the most common sinus tumour to invade the orbit. It typically causes superior displacement of the globe (upward dystopia; hyperglobus) as the tumour invades upwards through the floor of the orbit.

Encephalocoele is formed by herniation of intracranial tissues through a congenital defect of the base of the skull. It usually displaces the globe forward and downwards.

Optic nerve glioma and cavernous haemangioma are retrobulbar space-occupying lesions within the muscle cone that cause axial proptosis where there is a forward displacement of the globe.

94) B

The trochlear nerve emerges from the superior orbital fissure outside the annulus of Zinn (see explanation and diagram for Question 3 in Chapter 7).

95) D

Pseudophakic cystoid macular oedema (CMO), also known as Irvine-Gass syndrome, is one of the most common causes of visual loss after cataract surgery. It is believed to be caused by the breakdown of the blood-aqueous and blood-retinal barriers, secondary to the upregulation of inflammatory mediators following surgical manipulation. This, in turn, leads to increased vascular permeability and fluid accumulation in the outer plexiform and inner nuclear layers of the retina. Pre-existing diabetes confers an increased risk of developing pseudophakic CMO.

96) A
The inner mucin layer of the tear film is secreted by the conjunctival goblet cells, glands of Manz and the crypts of Henle.

97) C
The secondary actions of the right superior oblique are depression and abduction. It is therefore an agonist, rather than an antagonist, of right eye abduction.

98) A
The nasolacrimal duct opens into the inferior nasal meatus of the nasal cavity with an opening — the aperture of the nasolacrimal duct. The aperture is located beneath the inferior nasal concha and is partly covered by a flap-like mucosal fold called the valve of Hasner.

99) B
The structures traversing through the foramen ovale can be remembered using the mnemonic **MALE** (**M**andibular nerve, **A**ccessory meningeal artery, **L**esser petrosal nerve, **E**missary veins).

The table below summarises the main foramina of the skull (which you should be familiar with) and the structures that traverse them, as well as which cranial fossa they lie in.

Cranial Fossa	Foramen	Structures Passing Through
Anterior	Cribriform plate of ethmoid bone	CN I
Middle	Optic canal	CN II
	Superior orbital fissure	CN III, IV, V_1, VI
	Foramen rotundum	Maxillary nerve (V_2)
	Foramen ovale	**M**andibular nerve (V_3) **A**ccessory meningeal artery **L**esser petrosal nerve **E**missary veins
	Foramen spinosum	Middle meningeal artery
	Foramen lacerum	Pterygoid artery/veins Internal carotid artery

Posterior	Internal auditory meatus	CN VII, VIII
	Jugular foramen	CN IX, X, XI
	Hypoglossal canal	CN XII
	Foramen magnum	Spinal cord

CN: Cranial Nerve

100) C

Use the table below to help remember the different segments of the optic nerve and their corresponding lengths. The intraocular is the shortest and the intraorbital is the longest.

Portion	Length (mm)
Intraocular	1
Intraorbital	25–30
Intracanalicular	6
Intracranial	10

Lightning Source UK Ltd.
Milton Keynes UK
UKHW022029270421
382739UK00007B/45